Brittany's Rose

Finding Peace after Losing a Loved One

Mary Jane Clayton

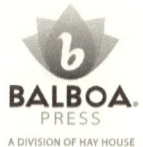

BALBOA.
PRESS
A DIVISION OF HAY HOUSE

Balboa Press books may be ordered through booksellers or by contacting:

Balboa Press
A Division of Hay House
1663 Liberty Drive
Bloomington, IN 47403
www.balboapress.com
1-(877) 407-4847

ISBN: 978-1-4525-5145-6 (sc)
ISBN: 978-1-4525-5147-0 (hc)
ISBN: 978-1-4525-5146-3 (e)

Library of Congress Control Number: 2012908034

Printed in the United States of America

Balboa Press rev. date: 06/25/2012

For my granddaughter,

Brittany Alex Engle

Our Sweet Angel

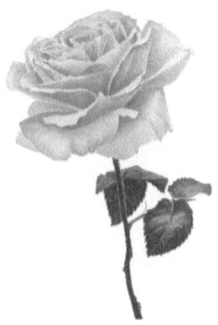

Also for my daughter, Lori, who listened to the message in spite of the pain, a message that led her to a life's work of teaching others how to have a healthy and happy life. Even though her heart was breaking, she was always my rock.

To Gary, Brittany's father, who struggled from afar as he learned of his daughter's illness early one morning in the sands of Saudi Arabia during the first Gulf War. After years of struggling through many great trials, he now leads a happy and successful life.

Acknowledgements

I thank God and my granddaughter Brittany who, from the windows of heaven, guided me through this emotional journey. The spirit of their love made it possible for love from the other side to reach our family and many others.

With all my heart, I thank my daughter, Lori, and Brittany's dad, Gary, for letting me tell their story. Their love gave me the courage to keep writing.

Thanks also to Alfred Music Publishing for giving me permission to use the song *The Rose* in this book. This song will forever be a symbol of Brittany's message.

I thank Ed Rivera and his wife for being at the church on the day I needed them. The two pink roses he painted will forever be a true testimony to how God works His magic.

Many thanks to my editor and project partner, Rene Seabaugh, for generously sharing his wisdom and believing in me as a writer.

A special thanks to my dear friend Diane Jacob for proofreading my manuscript and doing some additional editing.

Another special thanks to Rebecca Servoss who designed the cover and jacket of the book. Her divine talent gave it the perfect touch of heaven.

Contents

Why I Wrote This Book

I'm an ordinary person just like you, trying to keep up with life and make the most of every day. Usually, we wake up each morning with plans for what we need or want to do that day. We get ourselves in gear and begin to put the day's plan in motion without ever thinking life might throw us a curve ball. Then, one day, we get that pitch. While some curve balls may only require us to make a slight adjustment, others can leave us stunned. If you've ever received news that put you in a state of shock, you know how it feels to be left wondering how you can possibly handle what was just thrown your way.

This is the story of a little girl and the power of a pink rose. This little girl is my granddaughter, Brittany, who died of leukemia two weeks after her fifth birthday. After her passing, the weight of grieving was burying me alive. I needed to find a way to express what was going on inside me, and writing seemed to be the answer. I started my journal about a month after her passing. When I first began, I wrote anything and everything that came into my head. It was a way of releasing anger and sorrow without bothering anyone else. As I wrote, I realized I was still struggling to find answers to the many questions. I started and stopped more times than I can remember because writing about this loss required me to relive too many extremely confusing and heartbreaking moments.

During this time, there were periods when my faith and beliefs were greatly tested. I thought I knew what I believed in, but then realized I wasn't so sure. Confusion and anger held me back and kept me from moving through the grief. I knew I had to figure out what I truly believed in; otherwise, I had nothing to grasp on to, nothing to help pull me up and over the edge.

Over the years since Brittany's death, many events occurred that could easily be called coincidences. At first, I attributed these "coincidences" to wishful thinking, but as they continued to happen, my emotional connection to them became stronger. When I began to realize these events had the characteristics of a message, I became curious as to what these messages might be. I knew I had to start trusting my intuition and pay more attention to what went on around me or nothing would change. Surprisingly, the more I paid attention, the more I felt Brittany's presence.

Eventually, I stopped asking for proof that what I was experiencing was real, and started to just believe. This is when everything changed for me. Once I began believing, it became easier to understand the messages without the need for conscious reasoning. I no longer needed to question or justify my interpretation of these events because I knew I had become part of a divine connection.

Brittany was using these messages to show me that she was still close by. Her messages were meant to lift me up, warm my heart, and keep our memories alive.

The turning point for me was when I made the choice to believe in the unbelievable. As the pieces began coming together, I gradually moved toward a place of peace.

The loss my family experienced is not unique. It happens every day and will continue to happen. The purpose of this book is to share how my experiences helped me discover what I truly believed in. Only then was I able to accept this great loss.

As you move through this journey, I hope you will realize that those who have passed on are still within your reach. You just have to learn to touch them in a different way.

If you are still searching for peace of mind, I trust something you read will ring true to you. If not, I hope it will at least inspire you to look for new ways of finding answers.

Chapter One

Faith and Hope at Work

SCHOOL BEGINS

From the kitchen, I heard a squeak as the screen door slowly opened and closed. It wasn't the same sound as when the kids ran in and out. It sounded more like someone was "sneaking" in. Hum? I leaned around the corner to see who it was. There, standing quietly, with both hands behind her back and a sweet grin on her face, was my granddaughter, Brittany. She was just a little thing, not quite five, with long brown hair and big brown eyes just like her mother.

"I have something for you, Grandma," she said. I could tell by her smile she was excited to be bringing a surprise. With her hands still behind her back, she whispered, "Close your eyes." I knelt down to her level and closed my eyes.

"OK, open," she said, as a smile stretched across her face. There, clutched in her hands, were two fully bloomed pink roses. Her eyes beamed as she handed one to me and said the other was for her mom. I reached forward, pulled her in for a hug, and kissed her on the cheek. I love those unspoken words that live inside hugs.

I graciously accepted her gift with a polite, "Thank you, Sweetie. It's beautiful!"

We could hear my daughter, Lori, coming, so Brittany and I hurried and hid behind the wall. She looked at me with big eyes and put her finger over her lips to sign "Sh-h-h." We stood still, trying not to move or make a sound. It was fun feeling like a kid again. Lori walked right past us and didn't even know we were there. Brittany quietly peeked around the wall and waited until Lori had her back to us. Then, she ran out and said, "Mom!" Lori jumped about three feet from the ground.

Lori put her hands on her chest and said, "Good grief, why did you do that?" After we got all our laughs out, Brittany handed the rose to Lori.

As I watched, I remembered when I was little and what a big deal it was to give someone a surprise. It began with having someone you wanted to give a surprise to. That alone was something to be grateful for. Then, you got the idea for the surprise and planned how you would give it. The whole process brings its own unique type of joy.

"Oh, thank you, Sweetie," Lori said, as she leaned over and gave Brittany a big hug and kiss. "This is so beautiful! I think Grandma and I should put our flowers in a vase and put them on the dinner table."

"OK," Brittany said, jumping up and down. Lori found a vase with a narrow opening, filled it with water, and set it on the table. Brittany climbed onto the chair and carefully put the flowers in the vase before moving it to the center of the table.

"They sure make our table look beautiful," Lori said. Along with the beauty of the gift was the precious tiny hand of the giver.

Pink roses have always been Brittany's favorite. She had pink roses on pajamas, dresses, shoes, ribbons, shirts, and everything else. When Lori and I shopped, we always looked for things with pink roses on them and were always so happy when we found something. Do we ever outgrow the thrill of finding a "special gift" for someone we love?

In Southern California, some January mornings are just as warm and sunny as in summer, and that's how it was on this day. We were getting ready to go on an extra special shopping spree to buy new clothes for Brittany. The next day was to be her first day at a new preschool and she was excited about making new friends. Erik, Brittany's brother, who was just a year-and-a-half old, was going to spend time with Uncle Matt while we shopped.

As Lori and I quickly tidied up the house, Brittany and Erik played in the front room. Erik loved all the attention Brittany gave him. Earlier, he had toddled over to her, and as she opened her arms and hugged him, she said, "He's so lovable." Now that just warms your heart!

Lori gathered up what she needed for Erik, and I went to freshen up a bit. I asked Brittany to come with me so we could comb her hair. I lifted her up onto the bathroom counter so she could watch in the mirror. She liked having long hair and I loved combing it just like I did her mom's when she was little. She watched as I pulled the sides back to make a small ponytail near the top of her head. Then, for the final touch, I wrapped a ribbon with tiny pink roses on it around the ponytail. After fluffing her bangs, I put just a touch of hair spray on them.

Her little face beamed as she said, "Thank you, Grandma. That looks so pretty." I gave her a kiss on the cheek, moved her hair back off her shoulders, and helped her down.

"Oh, Grandma, wait. Can I put on some lip gloss?" she asked.

"Of course," I said, as I lifted her back up onto the counter. I smiled to myself as I watched her press her upper lip slightly against her teeth just the way her mother and I did when we put on our lipstick. For a second, I imagined her getting ready for her first prom. She rubbed the gloss on and moved her lips together with a back and forth motion to make sure it was spread evenly. She turned her head a little to the left and took one last glance in the mirror before climbing down.

"Are you guys ready?" Lori hollered down the hall.

"Yes," Brittany said, as she skipped toward the living room.

This was going to be quite an exciting day. Shopping for new school clothes is an adventure all its own. It's not the same as getting them for your birthday or Christmas. On this shopping spree, Brittany would get to pick everything out by herself, and even buy more than one pair of shoes!

Four hours later, we came home dragging bags and bags of clothes. As Brittany skipped back to her room with a couple bags, her soft hair bounced along behind her. With a few more bags hanging from my arms, I followed. While Lori was in the kitchen starting dinner, Brittany and I dumped all the clothes out on the bed. She put dresses on one side and matching tops and bottoms on the other. Next, she jumped up on the bed and lined up all the shoes neatly across the pillows. I smiled to myself as I tried to imagine what she must be thinking. After arranging everything in its place, she asked if she could do a fashion show. I was all for that, but first we had to have dinner.

Kicking off my shoes, I turned on some soft music and started setting the table. I really wanted to sit down and relax, but I knew how anxious Brittany was for dinner to be over so we could get on with the show. I have to admit, I ate kind of fast because I was excited to see how cute she would look all dressed up. We didn't have to pick Erik up for another hour so this would be a special time just for us girls. This was one of those moments when you stop and smell the roses.

For the next thirty minutes, Lori and I watched as Brittany modeled each outfit. Once, she came out wearing a cute plaid jumper and a different shoe on each foot. We weren't sure why until she put her hands on her hips, pointed one foot out and then the other and said, "Which shoe looks better with this outfit?"

Holding in our laughs, Lori and I looked at each other and smiled. It was such a sweet moment. Lori pointed to her left foot and said, "I think that one looks the best."

We watched as she paraded out in each new outfit and did a few modeling poses. It took a little longer than expected because she wanted to dress herself each time. When she was done, she took a little bow and made her exit. If only I'd had a video camera!

While Lori went to pick up Erik, I helped Brittany hang up her clothes and get ready for bed. After picking out what she wanted to wear to school, she put her PJs on and we went to the living room to watch TV. She climbed onto the couch beside me and laid her head in my lap. We were both exhausted from the day, and she could barely keep her eyes open. I began slowly running my fingers through her hair and pushing it away from her face.

After a few minutes, she started coughing and said her throat hurt. I didn't like hearing that because tomorrow was a big day, and she just couldn't get sick now. I quickly pushed the thought out of my head and decided that just wasn't going to happen. I gave her some Tylenol and sprayed her throat, hoping that would help her have a good night's rest. Her cheeks were warm, but not too bad. I was sure she'd be fine by morning.

Lori came home with Erik, who had fallen asleep on her shoulder. I told her Brittany was feeling a little sick and that I had given her some medicine. Brittany and I got up, and the four of us went down the hall to the kids' room. Lori got Erik into his PJs and tucked him in as I tucked Brittany in. I gave her a kiss on the cheek and a little tickle and said, "Nighty night, don't let the bed bugs bite." She laughed and said, "Good night, Grandma. I love you."

"I love you too, Sweetie Pie," I said, as I reached over and gave her toe a little squeeze through the blanket. I gave Erik a hug and a kiss, and left Lori to give them their goodnight hugs and kisses from mom.

Eventually, all the lights were out and everyone was safe in their beds. As I lay in mine, the cool night air crept into my room, giving me the feeling I was swinging in a hammock under the moonlight on some tropical island. The house was quiet, except for a cough now and then from Brittany's room.

The previous week, Lori had taken Brittany to see her new school and to meet her teacher. She got to see her classroom and where she would play with her new friends during recess. At home, we spent time talking with Brittany about new things she would learn, about the playground, and even what she would bring for lunch. Finally, the first day of school was only hours away. Mentally, I went over my list . . . the alarm clock was set, Brittany's lunch was made, the car had a full tank of gas, and I had decided what we were having for breakfast. I had a hard time falling asleep because I was so excited for it to be morning.

My alarm went off at 5:30 a.m., and, as usual, I turned on the TV to listen to the news. Every channel had news stories from the Middle East. We kept close tabs on those stories because Lori's husband, Gary, was in the Army in this war they called Desert Storm. As a medic, he got a close-up view of things we would never see. It was a tough job, both physically and emotionally.

His unit was the furthest deployed North Eastern American Unit based in Saudi Arabia. They provided medical support for the 1st Calvary as they built roads into Iraq. When the ground war began, they were attached to the 82nd Airborne Division, which was getting ready to head into Iraq.

Every day we prayed for all the men and women in harm's way, but almost daily, a family got bad news. The emotional strain was hard to cover up at times.

A few months earlier when Gary was preparing to leave home, I had asked Lori and the kids to come and stay with me while he was gone. Lori was only 23 years old and I knew it wouldn't be easy for her to take care of two small children by herself. Gary agreed it was a good idea, so a couple weeks before he deployed, he packed them up and moved them from Colorado to California.

As I was putting on my makeup, I realized Lori should have been up by now. After all, it was Brittany's first day at her new school. I didn't want her to be late, so I peeked in the bedroom to see if they were up and getting ready. I was surprised to see all of them sound asleep. In a panic, I nudged Lori and quietly said, "Lori, you need to get up." When she rolled toward me I could see her eyes were puffy and red. Her face had "worry" written all over it.

She sat up and put her hand on Brittany's head. "Mom," she said, "we've been up all night. She just barely fell asleep. I took her temperature and it went off the top of the thermometer. I can't take her to school like this. I have to call the doctor."

My heart sank. This was not how the day was supposed to be. I thought of calling work and telling them I wouldn't be in, but Lori said to go, and she would call me when they got home from the doctor. I squeezed Lori's hand, told her everything would be fine, and asked her to call me as soon as she learned something.

I kept telling myself not to worry, whatever is supposed to happen will happen, and we will work it out. It's not always easy to stay strong, but as a mother and grandmother, I felt it was my job to be a good example of a positive philosophy. Staying calm would show I had faith that God was watching over us. Of course, I worried anyway.

At about ten o'clock, Lori called me at work. I knew something was wrong because I heard a panic in her voice I had never heard before. She told me that by the time they got to the doctor's office, Brittany was burning up with fever. They had immediately called for an ambulance and she was taken to Children's Hospital in the city of Orange.

It took all Lori's strength to keep from breaking down as she told me they had to put Brittany in a tub of ice to get the fever down. I couldn't imagine how that must have felt. Even with a fever, it must have been terribly cold and painful. My heart ached as I thought of Lori listening to her child scream and watching helplessly as she begged to be pulled from the freezing water. I couldn't believe this was happening. I covered the receiver, took a deep breath and let it out, trying not to let Lori hear the fear in my voice.

Trying to stay calm, I asked, "What do they think is wrong?"

In a shaky voice she answered, "They don't know yet. They just took some blood and have to do some tests."

"It's probably just a touch of the flu," I said. "The doctors are being cautious. I'm sure she'll be fine in a couple days." She agreed and said she would call me later when she had more to tell.

"Lori," I asked, "is Erik with you?"

"No," she answered. "I called Matt and he was able to come and pick him up."

I was relieved to hear that and told her I would pick Erik up on my way home.

It was hard to keep my mind on work, but I was glad I had something to do. I tried to stay positive and concentrate, but every few minutes I thought of Lori and what was happening at the hospital. Sometimes, I would stop working and just stare at the phone, waiting for it to ring.

Around three o'clock, Lori finally called. All she said was, "Mom." Then there was a pause. I could hear the tears as she spoke that word and knew what she was going to tell me was not good news.

"What's wrong, Lori? How is Brittany?" I asked.

With a broken voice she said, "She has leukemia." Then she started to cry.

"Oh, Lori, are they sure?" I asked quickly.

"Yes," she answered through the tears.

I tried to sound positive as I told her, "Everyone at that hospital knows how to treat this disease. They'll take good care of her. She'll be OK. Just have faith." Even though I was doing my best to stay positive, I could feel the fear running through me.

When she didn't respond, I knew she was terrified. I wanted to burst into tears, but I couldn't do that. Not now.

"I'm leaving for the hospital," I said quickly. "I'll be there in twenty minutes."

I hung up the phone and just stood there. My legs were numb. I couldn't talk. I couldn't move. I couldn't look at anyone. During that moment, the fear of the unknown consumed me. I tried to pull my thoughts together and make sense of things, but it was impossible.

I had told my boss earlier about the night's events, so he knew it might be a rough day. He could tell something was wrong and came over to my desk. With a blank stare, I said, "I need to go to the hospital. Brittany has leukemia." He just stood there, speechless.

Finally he said, "Go, MJ, just go. Don't worry about anything here. Call if there is anything I can do." He gave me a hug and pushed me toward the door.

My mind was spinning as I tried to put together a plan to assure my daughter that everything was going to be OK, but before one thought was complete, another would start. It was almost impossible to think clearly. I kept imagining our sweet little Brittany shivering and thinking, "What's happening to me? Why does everyone look so worried? Why does my body feel so strange? Will I be able to go to school tomorrow?"

I got in my car and headed toward the freeway. Normally, the drive would only take about fifteen minutes, but traffic was a mess, which stressed me out because I wanted to get there quickly. As I looked around at all the cars, I wondered where people were going and how many of them had ever faced this kind of fear. Every day, people pack the freeways as they drive to and from someplace, but we know nothing about them. They're just people in cars on the road, and we have no idea what they might be dealing with. I began to wonder how many of them might be heartbroken today.

As my mind drifted to what was happening at the hospital, everything around me seemed to blend into a mesh of gray. An awful, unsettling feeling was weighing heavily on me and I didn't know how to shake free of it. I suppose it was natural to feel that way, but I knew it wouldn't comfort Lori if I walked in with a long, sad face. The closer I got to the hospital, the more frightened I became. Tears welled up in my eyes as I thought of seeing Brittany lying in a hospital bed.

As I wiped away the tears, I looked up at the sky in front of me. What I saw made me want to stop right there in the middle of the road. It seemed strange to be compelled to stop like that, but the feeling was so strong that I didn't question it. I looked for a safe place to pull over and made my way to the side of the road.

When I looked up again, a surreal feeling came over me as I stared at a beautiful patch of clouds with sunbeams spreading down and out like a giant fan. They covered the sky in front of me with a magical aura. Yes, it really did feel magical. As I watched in awe, I was completely taken in by the beauty of this moment. God was reaching out to me. I just knew it.

I reached forward and pressed my hand to the windshield. Through the glass, I felt God's hand reaching back to me. Each ray of light was like a finger of His hand, and for that moment, fear disappeared. I kept my hand pressed to the windshield, hanging on to the peaceful feeling as long as I could.

I felt lifted up and connected to God and all that ever was and will be. It was the right time for a whispered prayer.

"Thank you, God, for this new feeling of hope. Thank you for letting me know You will help us through whatever lies ahead."

I became determined to show faith in a way I had never shown it before. As I took the final exit toward the hospital, I pictured exactly what would happen. I would walk in with such a positive attitude that everything would change. Brittany's temperature would be normal and she would be sitting up, smiling. The doctor would give her some medicine and we would all go home. Then we would lay out what she was going to wear to school. At the dinner table, we would talk about how much fun her first day of school was going to be. Later, Lori would tuck the kids into bed and we would all put our heads on our pillows and happily drift into peaceful sleep.

After parking the car, I got out and stood still for a moment. As I stared ahead, all I could think was . . . in front of me stood a building filled with sick children and scared parents. This was a world I knew nothing about. My feet felt glued to the ground. Neither foot wanted to be the one to take the first step.

The elevator doors opened to the second floor. As I stepped out, a nurse pulling a wagon was passing by. In the wagon was a little girl with no hair, about four years old, hooked up to an IV. She looked up and smiled at me as they passed. I meant to smile back, but I'm not sure if I did. Sadness pressed hard on my heart and for those few seconds, I felt completely disconnected from everything. I kept saying, "Brittany does not belong here. No child belongs here. Why does this happen?" At that moment, the reality of my granddaughter being in a life threatening situation struck me, and it struck hard.

As I walked down the hall, I couldn't help peeking into the rooms. It was heartbreaking to see all the children with no hair. Some were lying still, some were talking with their families, and some had doctors and nurses gathered around their beds. The thought of becoming part of all this was more than I could comprehend.

Room 215 . . . there it was. Before walking in, I took in a deep breath and slowly blew it out. Doing this always helped me gain control of my mental state. Lori was sitting on the edge of Brittany's bed holding her hand. When Lori saw me, she got up and walked over to me. As I reached out and put my arms around her, my teeth were tightly pressed together as I struggled not to cry. I could feel the burning in my throat. For a moment, we just held each other because neither of us could speak.

Caught off guard and in complete disbelief, we wondered what to reach out and grab on to. Emotions we'd never dealt with before were swallowing us whole. We told ourselves this couldn't be happening, but it was. The world we knew just a few hours ago was now all mixed up.

Brittany looked completely exhausted as she lay quiet and still. When I leaned over to give her a kiss on the cheek, I saw how tired her eyes looked. I had never seen her like that. I brushed her hair back from her forehead and smiled at her.

"You've had a rough day, haven't you, Sweetie," I quietly said. Too weak to speak, she slowly nodded her head.

Lori hadn't eaten all day, so I told her I would sit with Brittany while she went and got a bite, and we could talk when she came back. I knew she needed a break, and that she wanted to make some phone calls to let everyone know what was going on.

One of her most important calls was to the Red Cross. Surely they would know how to contact Brittany's dad, Gary, and have him sent home. She called and told them what was happening; giving them all the information she had about where Gary might be. They told her they weren't sure how long it would take to contact him, but that they would start working on it right away. I don't know how the Red Cross finds someone on the battlefield, but that is part of their job. We had faith they would find him soon and send him home.

Many of our relatives lived out of state, so the phone was kept busy with updates. Like the rest of us, they couldn't believe what was happening. They kept asking, "She'll be all right, won't she?" Even those who were nearby didn't visit the first day because they thought she would be coming home that night or in the morning.

While Lori was making calls, I pulled a chair close to the bed and laid my head beside Brittany's pillow. I took her hand and rubbed my thumb back and forth across her little fingers. I closed my eyes and asked God to send his healing power to her small body.

> *"God, she's just a tiny thing and doesn't know what's happening to her. If she did, I know she would fight hard to get better. We feel so helpless and don't know what to do. Please help us understand what we can do to make her better."*

I repeated the prayer again and again.

After a while, she opened her eyes and turned her head toward me. It was easy to see she was physically drained. I tried to think of something to talk about that would sound positive. She knew I was trying to lose weight, so I said, "Guess what?"

"What?" she answered in almost a whisper.

"I lost four more pounds! Soon I'll be able to run a race with you and I might even win!" I laughed as I spoke, hoping to get a smile from her.

She looked me straight in the eyes and said in a tiny whisper, "Grandma, I love you just the way you are." I clenched my teeth and drew a deep breath in through my nose. I wanted to burst into tears and hug her so tight. Her eyes closed, and she lay silent again. Oh, boy. This wasn't going to be easy. I just wanted to scoop her up and take her home.

I tried to think of something else to talk about, but since I could see it would be a strain for her to have a conversation, I just hummed some music and rubbed her hand. I laid my head down on the bed next to her cheek and closed my eyes.

About twenty minutes later, a soft pat on my shoulder woke me. Lori pulled up a chair and sat down. I asked her if she had any news from the doctors, but there was nothing new. Waiting was so difficult. We tried to think of only the positive, but worrying about what we might hear was so frightening that it was hard to keep the negative from creeping in.

It had been a long and emotional day, and I knew Lori was beat and needed to stretch out and rest. Brittany had been given something to help her sleep and was out for the night. Earlier, one of the nurses had rolled in a cot so Lori could stretch out and stay close to Brittany.

"Do you want me to stay with you tonight?" I asked.

She hugged me and said, "I'll be OK. Thanks, Mom. You don't need to stay. I'll see you in the morning."

I hugged her and said, "You be sure to call me, no matter what time it is, if you need me."

As I walked out the door, I turned back and took one last look into the room. Lori had just stretched out on the cot and was laying her head on the pillow. My heart hurt for her. This was such a heavy load to bear.

On my way home, I picked Erik up from Matt's house. Once we got home and had a little bite to eat, I got him ready for bed. He was an easy child to care for. He always did what he was told without fussing much. After picking out one of his favorite books, we snuggled in his bed and got comfortable. As I read, his little head fell farther and farther into my lap until he finally fell asleep. I slide out of bed and pulled the covers up over him and tucked him in.

After getting comfortable, I called my sister and my two brothers to let them know what was going on. They were quite taken back by this news. When people are so far away, it's hard for them to know what to do. There isn't much they can do other than listen and offer their support.

My mother was a world traveler and was somewhere on the other side of the planet. I hadn't heard from her in a while and had no idea where she was or when she would return. My father had passed away a year earlier. I really missed having his shoulder to lean on. I kept thinking that because he was in heaven, he could somehow help God make Brittany better.

Angels in Disguise

The next morning, I arranged for one of our neighbors to watch Erik during the day. She had a son about his age who was excited for Erik to come and play. This would be much easier than trying to keep him entertained at the hospital.

Soon, there I was again, walking down the hospital hallway peeking into the rooms of sick children and their families. Each family had their own story. Each family was in pain and afraid of what was to come. This was only one hospital out of hundred. So many of us live our lives without ever knowing the pain so many people are going through.

When I reached Brittany's room, Lori was sitting on the bed talking with her. I could tell Brittany had probably slept well because the head of the bed was raised and they were watching TV. She usually didn't like watching TV so much.

After giving her a kiss on the cheek, I said, "You look like you feel better."

"Not really," she whispered.

As I brushed my hand softly across her check, I said, "I know it's hard right now, but you'll feel better soon."

I asked Lori, "Have you heard anything from the doctors this morning?"

"Nothing yet," she replied. "It's so hard to sit here and wait to hear about all these tests. I'm not even sure what all they are testing for. Mom, can you sit with Brittany for a while? I have something I need to do."

"Sure I will. Where are you going?"

"I need to find some help, Mom. I need to find someone who can help us."

I wasn't sure what she meant, but I told her to go ahead. This wasn't the time to ask questions. I knew I needed to just let her go and do whatever it was she needed to do. I could see she was in panic mode. I worried about her emotional state, but Lori was strong, so I had to trust she knew what she was doing.

I got out a coloring book and some crayons and Brittany and I each picked a favorite picture to color. I picked a little dragon and asked Brittany what color I should make him.

"He should be green," she said.

"OK, then. He will be green." She picked a little girl swinging on a swing. I watched as she took a yellow crayon and carefully colored her curly hair. Talking seemed to take too much energy, so we just colored in silence. After a few minutes, she started nodding off so I took the book and crayons and lowered her bed so she could rest. I sat down and pulled another chair close so I could rest my feet. My eyes closed as I laid my head against the back of the chair. I couldn't stop wondering where Lori was and what she was doing. She had said she needed to find someone who could help, but what did that mean?

When Lori returned a couple hours later, she seemed much more at ease, making me curious about where she had gone.

"You look relieved, Lori. Did you find someone to help?" I asked.

"Well, I went to a New Age store near our house hoping to find someone who did energy healing work. While I was talking to the woman behind the counter, a man came up behind me and tapped me on the shoulder. He had been standing close by and overheard our conversation. He said he knew someone who could help and gave me the phone number of a woman named Barbara Bullard. I can't believe it, Mom. I found someone to help!"

I could only respond, "It was meant to be. Things like that don't just happen." It was wonderful to see her smile. I wasn't sure what to expect, but I knew a prayer had been answered and it felt good.

Lori looked at me and said, "I want to call her now."

"You go call," I told her. "I'll sit with Brittany."

Thankfully, Barbara was home when Lori called. Lori began by telling her how she had gotten her phone number and went on to tell her what was happening with Brittany. Barbara told her that not only did she do energy healing work, but she also used a technique called the Hemi-Sync procedure. This method consists of playing numerous audio tapes that work with specific sound waves and tones that lead the brain through various states in order to synchronize its two hemispheres. The program is designed to heal the mind, body, and soul at a deep level. Lori didn't understand it completely, but was willing to try anything that might help her little girl.

Barbara told Lori that she had two friends who also did energy healing: Kat Carroll, who, along with Barbara, was an instructor at Orange Coast College, and Dawn Ahart, who ran her own Holistic Health Center. All this was much more than Lori had expected. The weight of a thousand pounds was lifting from our shoulders. I asked Lori when they would be stopping by. She said maybe that day or that night. It may have been wrong to expect a miracle, but we did. Lori asked for help and there, delivered right in her hands, were Barbara, Kat, and Dawn.

Once you ask for what you need,
the secret is to believe it will happen.

About an hour later, Lori received a call from Dawn Ahart. She told Lori that Barbara had contacted her and said she would be coming that evening. As they talked, Dawn went on to explain what her Health Center did to help heal people, and that healing energies produced by one's self or person-to-person could be as effective as conventional medicine. This was commonly called "laying on of hands healing," even though hands did not always have to touch the body to be effective.

I'd never been involved with that kind of work, but Lori had studied in this area and understood it much better than I did. That's why she went looking for this kind of help. When someone's life is in danger, you reach out to anyone or anything that might be able to save them. You don't need to understand it completely. You just have to have faith and give it a chance. Knowing these women were there to help made it easier for us to relax a little.

Brittany was awake and wanted to sit up and color, so I decided to go back to work for a couple hours and give Lori and her some alone time. When I got to work, I gave my boss an update on the latest developments. He told me not to worry and to go back to the hospital whenever I needed to. He was a down-to-earth and kind-hearted person, and it was hard for him not to be able to do more to help. After taking care of a few things, I went back to the hospital.

While driving, I wondered if I would meet any of these women that night. Even though I didn't understand what they were going to do, my hope that they would make Brittany well was high. Healers heal people, right? Yes, I was expecting a miracle. I had a lighter step in my walk and I was even smiling as I entered the hospital.

As I reached Brittany's room, I saw a woman talking with Lori. I had never seen her before and she wasn't dressed like a nurse, so I assumed she was one of the women we were expecting. I put on my best smile and walked over to her.

"Mom," Lori said, "This is Dawn Ahart. She's one of the women I told you about earlier. She owns the Holistic Health Center."

As we shook hands, I could feel her calming energy. She was petite, well dressed and, in my eyes, beamed of heavenly light. Her smile drew me in immediately, and I felt great comfort in her presence. She told Lori and me to take a break so she could sit with Brittany and get to know her. Brittany took to her right away and seemed to enjoy having someone new to talk to. For the first time, we felt it was all right to leave for a little while. We did need a break, so off we went to the cafeteria. As we ate, we talked about how these women were going to help.

When we returned to the room, Brittany was sleeping soundly. It was comforting to see her looking so peaceful, just like she did when she was home in her own bed. I wanted to know what this really meant. How many healing sessions does it take to heal someone? If Dawn does this healing every day, how long before we can take Brittany home?

Here is Dawn's description of her first visit with Brittany:

"She was so small and frail. I could feel her love energy and that of all those who were by her side and attending to her in the hospital. Her temperature was elevated at the time, as she struggled against the infection that fought to invade her weakened body. As I began to do the "laying on of hands," her elevated temperature subsided. I stayed with her a little longer, knowing from experience that a one-time treatment may not hold. As the next thirty or forty minutes passed, I could feel her body heat increase and did another treatment. Again, her temperature returned to normal and she fell into a calming sleep."

Because of Dawn's nursing background, she was able to help explain what was going on. Having someone like this come into our lives so quickly was astonishing. I didn't know exactly what was happening, but we were hopeful and able to smile again.

Later that evening, Barbara Bullard came by. Along with three Hemi-Sync tapes, she brought an unwavering confidence in what she had to offer. She was soft spoken and radiated a feeling of assurance. Barbara explained that the tapes contained seven layers of brain waves at different frequencies, accompanied at times by soothing music. She had brought a variety so that she could find the ones that worked best for Brittany.

When Brittany woke up, Lori introduced Barbara and told her Barbara had some nice music for her to listen to. To our surprise, but not Barbara's, Brittany was immediately receptive to this. She put the headphones on and lay back as if she knew exactly why she was listening to the tapes. Somehow, it made all of us more relaxed. Some of the nurses asked about the tapes because they noticed a difference when they walked into the room. They too felt the calming effect. As you can imagine, our spirits were greatly lifted by this.

That night, we also got to meet Kat Carroll. Kat had a smile as big as all outdoors. She was also soft spoken, but a little spunkier, and full of positive energy. Kat did Reiki energy healing work, as did Barbara. Again, not knowing exactly what to expect, Lori and I were ready to listen and learn. We were surprised when Kat told us, "You know, just a couple weeks ago, I put a message out to God asking Him to give me something to work on, and here I am, helping your beautiful family."

Kat didn't want to overwhelm Brittany on her first visit, so we all just sat and chatted while Brittany listened to one of the tapes. It was good to have this time to get to know each other. Kat could tell we were scared and desperately searching for help. I didn't understand what Reiki healing was about, so I asked Kat to tell me a little about it.

She said it is used to harmonize and balance the body physically, mentally, emotionally, and spiritually. The person performing the treatment can lay their hands on the person or they can just hold their hands over them. Then they channel what they call the "universal energy" through their body and to the person they are working on. The energy automatically flows to where it is needed.

That night, she and Barbara both did some Reiki healing while Brittany slept. They stood at the sides of her bed and pointed their palms toward her. It looked like they were meditating, but they were bringing healing energy from the universe to her. Surprisingly, it seemed to have a calming effect on anyone who entered the room. It was quite amazing and gave us a new wave of inspiration and hope.

The three women we met that day were ready for an assignment, so to speak, and the doors opened up for all of us. From that day on, one or two of them were there with us every day. They were there to help us, and we were there to help them fulfill their purpose. For us to find them, all three of them in one day . . . well . . . how often would something like that happen? It was no coincidence. It was God's hand choosing us all for a learning experience we would never forget.

Reality Hits

The day came when it was time to start Brittany's chemotherapy treatment. There was no more hoping the diagnosis was wrong. We knew it was happening, but accepting the truth was still difficult. How did this come about so quickly?

When I got to Brittany's room that day, I saw that her bed was empty. Then I saw Lori sitting quietly in the corner staring out the window. I ran to her.

"Lori, where is Brittany?" I asked, as I quickly sat down next to her.

She looked at me and quietly explained, "They took her to put a tube in her chest to give her intravenous chemotherapy. It's called a broviac. It's a rubber tube that's tunneled under her skin a short way from where it goes in the central artery just above her heart. They stitch it in place and cover it with a dressing so they can administer the chemo and any other medication. She'll have a short tube hanging from her chest. This way, she's not attached to the IV bag all the time."

"Oh, my," I sighed. "They knocked her out to do that, didn't they?"

"Yes," Lori answered. "Of course they did."

"Oh, Lori, I just can't believe this." I put my arms around her and pulled her to me. She cried softly as we sat without talking.

"Mom," Lori said, "how am I going to do this? I just don't know how I'm going to do this."

I hugged her tightly and said, "We'll figure it out. Don't worry. We'll do whatever it takes because we have to." This was a lot for even the strongest person, but all the other families with children there at the hospital had to deal with this same uncertainty and worry. We all had to struggle through it somehow.

We didn't want Brittany to see fear in our faces and we didn't want her to know how sick she was. We always talked as if she would get better soon. We told her the treatments would make her better, but you could see she was confused. There were so many needles and so many tests. She had no idea what was happening. Sometimes she would ask when she could go home, and we would say, "Soon. We'll be going home soon."

That afternoon, I called my sons and told them it was time to come to visit. When they arrived, they paused at the doorway looking in. Shock was written clearly on their faces. As I looked at them, I remembered feeling the same way the first time I stood in that doorway. I motioned for them to come in and met them halfway. I gave them both a hug, and we walked over to Brittany's bed. She looked up at them and smiled.

"Guess what I have?" Ryan said, as he smiled down at her.

"What?" Brittany replied. Her eyes opened a little wider.

From behind his back, he pulled out her favorite teddy bear. Her arms slowly reached up as Ryan handed it to her. She took the bear and pulled it to her chest. After softly kissing it on the face, she snuggled it under her chin. What an emotional lift it was to see her smile. The boys did their best to make conversation by talking about things they would do when she got home, but I could see confusion in their faces. They didn't know how to process what was happening.

I understood what my sons were experiencing. The older you get, the more you see what can and does happen to people. You become much more conscious of the fact that life isn't fair and can change in an instant. Your first experience of those facts is usually the hardest. Things that once only existed in your mind become real. No matter how strong your beliefs are, no one is ever prepared for the overwhelming weight of emotions that engulf you when you are faced with the possibility of losing a loved one. That afternoon I realized that some of our most significant experiences happen when we are most afraid because our fear forces us to step out of our normal ways of thinking and search for understanding. As hard as it is, we need to have patience and give ourselves time to live the experience and believe the understanding will come.

After about twenty minutes, the boys and I walked out in the hall so I could update them with the latest information. I explained, "The doctors said she has the kind of leukemia they have the most success with."

Still concerned, they asked, "So, she's going to be all right?"

All I could say was, "I think so. What they've told us so far makes me think she will get through this." It was impossible to think otherwise.

They went back in the room and sat with Brittany. She seemed to like talking more that night and was even laughing a little.

As I sat and watched, I remembered all the times Brittany, her mom, and I had gone to the park to feed the ducks.

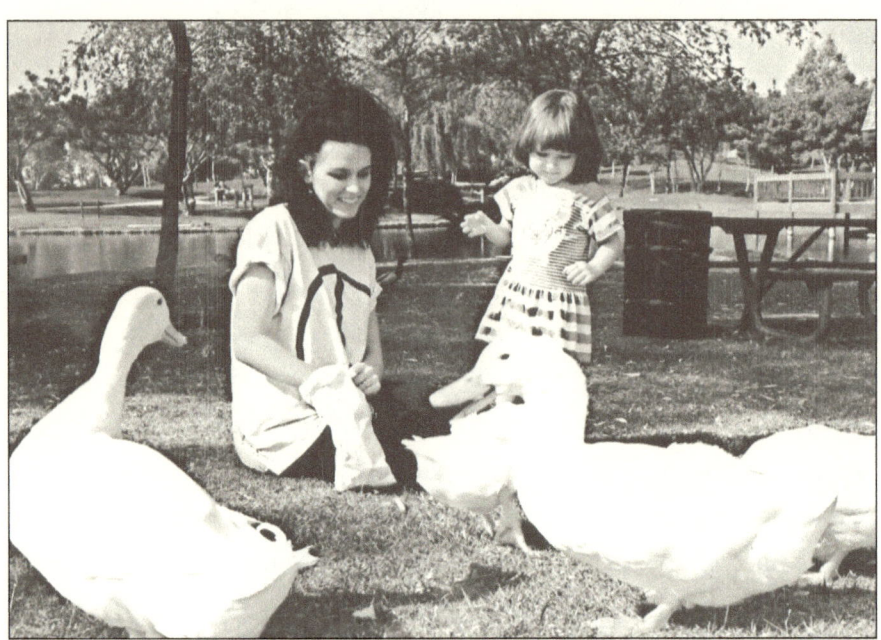

Brittany loved chasing the ducks. She would run slightly bent over with her arms stretched out in front of her hoping to catch one. Of course, she never did, but she kept running anyway, giggling joyfully the entire time. Her hair bounced up and down as her little feet ran faster and faster. It was so fun to watch. When she finally ran out of steam, we would get out the bread and all the ducks would come and huddle around to snatch bites from the ground. At those times in the park, we never hurried. Nature has a way of connecting you to the beauty and peacefulness of life, and we always took time to enjoy that.

Those outside the family, like Kat, Barbara, and Dawn, had never gotten to see the joyous side of Brittany. Some days while she was sleeping, Lori would describe to the women what she was like as a healthy child. They enjoyed hearing about her and connecting with who she was. The more they knew of her, the easier it was for them to do their work.

HELP FROM THE RED CROSS

On the days I went to work, I called every hour to see if Lori had heard anything new. I wasn't surprised to hear the chemo was making Brittany sick, because the hospital staff had told us that would probably happen. Lori's voice broke as she told me how hard it was to just sit, watching Brittany get sicker and sicker, and not be able to do anything about it. Her emotional strength was being crushed by all the uncertainty.

One day during this period, I called and found Lori unusually troubled.

"Lori, you sound upset. What's wrong?" I asked.

I could hear the panic in her voice as she said, "Mom, the Army called this morning and said they were having a hard time finding Gary because it was difficult communicating with some of the people in the field. That just doesn't make sense. There's a war going on. They have to communicate!"

Hearing that bothered me, too, but I tried my best to calm her down. "Lori," I said, "Don't worry. They'll find him. Just give it a little more time. They'll find him because they have to."

"Operation Desert Storm" they called it. Who thinks of these names? War itself is so frightening, but to call the U.S. involvement in that war "Desert Storm" sounded terrifying. Since Gary was a medic, he saw firsthand what war can do. How would he ever erase those memories?

Like so many other families, we prayed every day for the safety of all the men and women in harm's way. Every day we hoped our loved one was safe. Every day our heart cried for the families that got bad news, and every day we prayed the next phone call would not be the one that devastated us. All we could do was wait to hear from the Red Cross.

As it turned out, we didn't have much longer to wait. Later that afternoon, a nurse peeked in and motioned for us to come out to the hallway. Since she was smiling, we hoped she had good news.

She spoke softly as she said, "The Red Cross just called and said Gary would be arriving in a couple days."

Tears filled my eyes as I moved toward Lori and said, "He's coming home, Lori! I told you they would find him." I hugged her and held her for a moment as the tears trickled down our faces. We looked at the nurse, whose eyes were as wet as ours, and said, "Thank you." She smiled back and gave us a thumbs-up.

Lori dried her eyes and walked back into the room to sit on the edge of Brittany's bed. Taking Brittany's hand she said, "Guess what, Sweetie. Daddy's on his way home and he'll be here in a couple days!"

Brittany's eyes lit right up. It's amazing what great medicine a piece of good news can be. I wanted so much for this moment to last forever. We all felt relieved to know he was safe and on his way home. It made it much easier for Lori and Brittany to enjoy their conversation that afternoon.

Even though her dad was far away in the war, Brittany would get a letter from him about once a week with pictures of his surroundings. On the days she got a letter, she would draw a picture and send it back to him. She didn't understand what war was about, but his letters assured her he was safe and that her Daddy thought about her all the time.

In one letter, he had written about a big spiny lizard he kept on a leash in front of the aid station. He described the lizard as about five feet long and a little scary looking. His pictures made everything come alive. She could see his laundry in a bucket along with pictures of tents and camels. These pictures and letters kept the two of them close while he was away.

dear Britt,

How are you? I got some
really nice drawings in the
mail yesterday. I really,
really really like them. I
hope you send more fun
stuff. Maybe mom will
take pictures of you, baby
brother, and her? I sure
hope so. See you later
— love Dadio

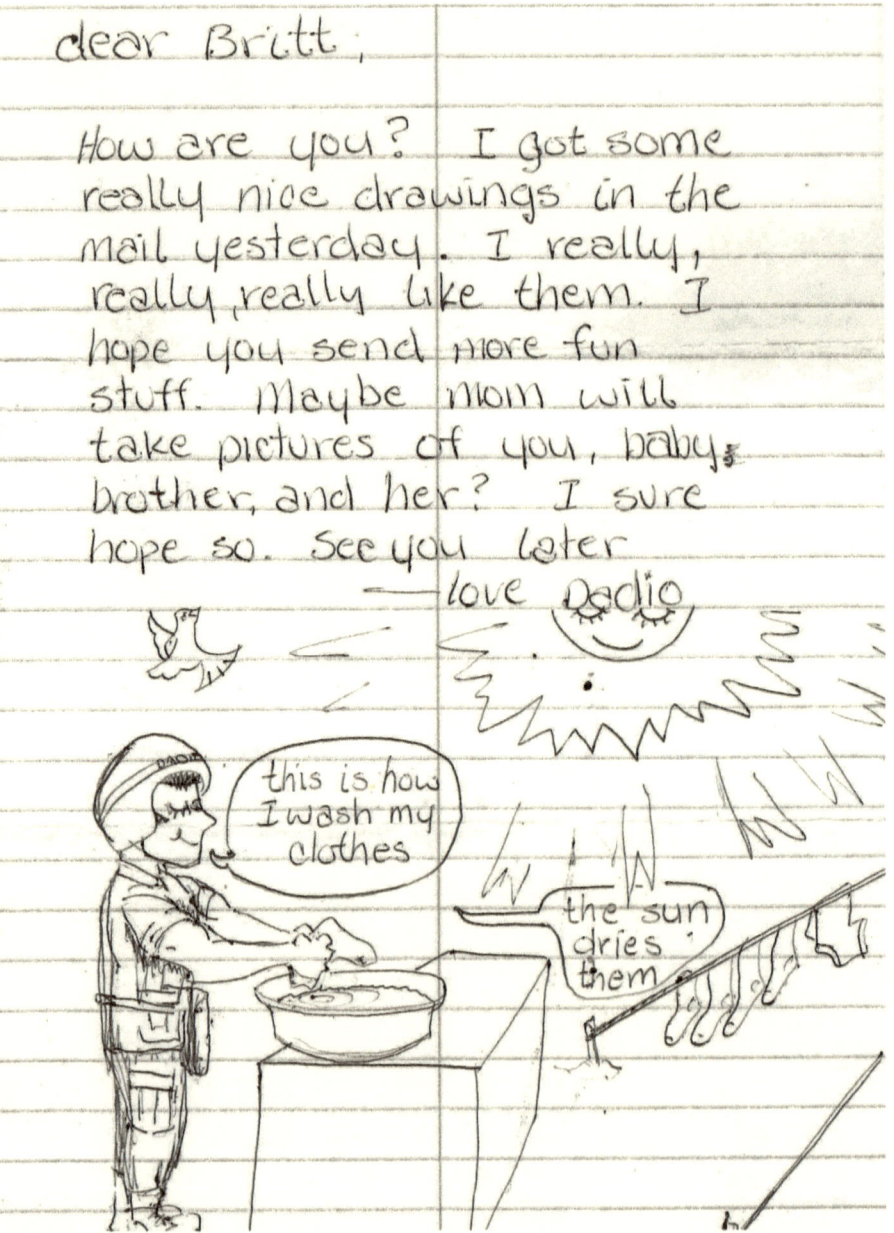

His letters to Lori were not the same as those to Brittany. As a medic, his job was to put people back together and keep them alive. As you can imagine, this could take an emotional toll on a person. In one letter he wrote:

> *"I would fall to sleep at night to the sounds of bombs rattling the earth. Bombers would fly by at about 200 feet elevation then drop the payload minutes later. We were protected by a single squadron of English fighter helicopters. One tank could have taken out our whole unit."*

I tried to picture how the Red Cross found him. Where was he when they told him? Was he sleeping, eating, or hunkered down somewhere in the sands of Saudi Arabia? Later he told us:

> *"In the early morning, before mail call, about 4:00 a.m., I was handed a letter. It was an offer for compassionate reassignment to Irvine, California. All it told me was Brittany had been admitted to the hospital. That was it. There was no mention of why. The next morning, I was on a C140 headed back to the States with nothing but a small backpack and my helmet."*

It's a long journey from the Middle East, but Gary was finally on his way. I imagined him sitting on the plane and wondered what must be going through his mind. How was he handling this? One day you're in a war, far away from your family, and then your child gets critically ill. Then suddenly you're on your way back home. It all seemed so unreal. You know this must happen every day to other families, but the reality that this time it's your family is so hard to accept.

Just having a solider come home from war was emotional enough, but to know he was leaving the battlefield because his child was diagnosed with an illness that could take her life . . . that was heartbreaking. We wondered if Brittany was in fact saving Gary's life by bringing him home. How would we ever know for sure?

The Wagon Ride

The previous day had been extremely hard on Brittany, so they had given her something to help her sleep through the night. After having a well-needed night of good rest, she seemed to be doing a little better. Lori sat on the side of the bed, gently brushing through her hair.

The door opened, and a nurse came in and asked if we would like to take her for a ride. I could see the handle of a wagon in the hallway. Emptiness rushed through me as I remembered the little girl in the wagon I had seen the first day I came to the hospital. I turned and looked to my daughter for an answer because I couldn't speak. I didn't want to put Brittany in that wagon.

Lori motioned for the nurse to bring it in. When Brittany saw the wagon, she was excited because it meant she could get out of bed. It wasn't easy, but Lori and the nurse managed to get her in the wagon. At least we were trying something new that might cheer her up.

Being able to take her for a ride seemed like progress, but I felt a rush of sadness when we had to prop her up with pillows and wondered if this was a good idea. I hadn't realized how weak she was. Brittany hadn't known it herself, and it made me sick to think how she must have felt when she realized she wasn't able to do this on her own. Her head lay back against the pillows, and her eyes stared ahead with little expression. Lori pulled the wagon and I walked behind. It was such a sad sight. I wanted to turn and run the other way and pretend it wasn't real. This isn't how a wagon ride should be. We should be having fun. Every day Lori tried to see and show only the bright side, but I knew, deep inside, she was terribly frightened.

People would pass by the wagon and say hello and we would nod back and smile. Lori did her best to make it fun. She was willing to do anything that might make Brittany feel like a healthy little girl again.

We went down a floor and out into a small garden. We followed the walkway until we found a little patio filled with flowers. As Brittany stared ahead, I wondered if she was thinking about our days at the park when she would run and play. We tried to have some conversation, but she didn't talk much. It seemed she was far away in another place. We weren't enjoying it like we thought we would, so we only stayed in the garden for a few minutes.

When we returned to the room, the nurse had to help us get her back into bed. It hurt her to be moved and going up instead of down was more of a strain on her body. I got the feeling she wouldn't want to get out of bed again and it broke my heart to think this might be as good as it would get. Once Brittany was settled again, I could see the pain in Lori's eyes as she realized how hard that little wagon ride had been.

About ten minutes later, a nurse brought in a pill for Brittany to take. Most of the medications were intravenous, but some needed to be taken by mouth. When the nurse tried to give Brittany the pill, she closed her mouth tight and turned away. After a moment, she turned her head back around and said in her tiny voice, "My daddy's a doctor. When he gets here, he'll help me take my medicine." Well, that was that, so they had to figure a way to put it in the IV. It quickly made her sleepy, and the nurse suggested we take a break while she slept. We got Gary's flight information from the nurses' station and went to the cafeteria to make plans for picking him up the next day.

That evening I went home early and let Lori have Brittany to herself. No one can make you feel as good as your mom and they needed some time alone. I kissed them both goodnight and left. On my drive home and for the next couple of hours I never stopped praying.

"Dear God, please take my dear Lori in your arms and hold her tight. She's so lost and so scared. You know she's a strong and brave person, but this time she needs Your help. She needs to rest just for a moment so please let her lay her head on Your shoulder. Our little Brittany is strong and brave just like her mother, but I know she doesn't understand what's happening. Kiss her cheek and help her to not be afraid. Thank You for my family and all those that are here for us. Help us to not lose faith, and bring her daddy home safely."

A Teacher's Precious Gift

Tragedy always brings people together, and that's what was happening to all of us at Children's Hospital. We had learned the names of the other parents and their kids. Instead of just passing by, we stopped and said hello and asked how things were going. We became a part of a community of people who knew what it was like to fight for your life. We shared hugs, hope, and prayers. We became more caring and patient, and developed a better sense of what's important and what isn't. Maybe all these little children were angels that came here to teach us and help us appreciate life more.

When I arrived that day, I was surprised by what I saw when I walked into Brittany's room. Handmade Get Well cards covered the wall that faced her bed. I could tell they were drawn by children, but who were they from?

"Wow, Brittany! Where did all these cards come from?" I asked, as I took a closer look.

Her little voice answered, "My friends at my new school drew them for me."

"My goodness, look at how many new friends you have. I wonder how many there are? Let's count them."

I pointed to each card as we counted until we reached fourteen. Earlier, Lori and Brittany had looked at them together before hanging them on the wall. They were from the kids that would have been her classmates at her new school. By now, she probably would have had a best friend.

I walked over to her bed and kissed her on the cheek and said, "Wow, with that many Get Well cards, I think you're going to get well really fast." She smiled just enough for it to be noticeable, but that was enough to do our hearts good. What a lovely gift this was from a caring teacher and her class.

I imagined the teacher telling the kids about Brittany and explaining what they were going to do to cheer her up. I pictured them thinking of her as they each created their special little card. I couldn't help wondering what Brittany was thinking as Lori hung each picture on the wall. She was supposed to be there with them— coloring, running, and playing.

I put my arm around Lori and said, "What a sweet thing to do."

"I know," she said, "I couldn't believe it when I opened the envelope and saw all these cards. I called the school today and thanked her."

Life is about people and that will never change. Deeds of kindness come from the heart. This was one of those times where the giver and the receiver shared the same joy.

Daddy's Coming Home

All day long, Brittany watched the hands on the clock as she counted the hours until her dad would be home. Gary's flight was to arrive in Los Angeles around seven o'clock that night. When you're anxious for something to happen, the hours seem to pass so slowly. No tests were scheduled, so Lori and Brittany spent the time coloring and watching TV. It was a long day of waiting, but finally, through the window, we could see the sun going down.

We were about an hour away from LAX, and it was time to go. Since Brittany was awake, I told Lori I would pick Gary up. This would give them some time to plan for his arrival. Lori is such a loving mother. She and Brittany were like two peas in a pod. Pretty much all their time together was quality time. It was easy to see the closeness they all shared.

I gave Lori a hug and walked over to Brittany's bedside, kissed her cheek, and told her I was on my way to the airport to pick up her daddy. Her eyes sparkled as she smiled from ear to ear. If she had been stronger, I know she would have jumped up and down on the bed saying, "Daddy's coming home! Daddy's coming home!" To see her look this happy was exhilarating.

As I drove, I imagined how anxious Gary must be to see his little girl. Since we hadn't had any direct communication with him, he didn't know what he was walking into. He knew she had been taken to the hospital, but he wasn't aware that she was still there.

Before I knew it, I had arrived at the airport. I parked the car and started walking to the terminal. Times had changed and now, no one was allowed to greet people as they came off the plane. Now, we had to wait behind the barrier.

There were about twenty of us waiting behind a barrier. Ahead, we saw a group of people coming toward us. This was the only plane arriving at this time, so I was sure he would be among them. Then I saw him, right in the middle of the group. My focus was on him and no one else. Everything outside that vision was blurred. There was a silence, as if the world had been put on pause for a moment.

Gary was easy to spot because he was the only one dressed in camouflage. He had a small backpack on his back, his helmet under his arm, and mud still on his boots. It was like something out of a movie. Once the group got closer, those waiting with me noticed there was a soldier in the crowd, and they all started clapping and cheering. My heart swelled with pride and sorrow at the same time. Tears filled my eyes, tears for a soldier coming home safe, and tears for what he was about to face. I walked toward him with open arms and welcomed him home.

"It's so good to have you home, Gary," I said, as I squeezed him tight.

He squeezed me back and said, "It's good to be home." I could tell he felt relieved to have his feet on the ground in a safe and familiar place.

I think "mellow" is a good way to describe Gary. He was always good at rolling with the punches, but I couldn't help but wonder what seeing the condition of his daughter would do to him.

We called Lori to let her know the plane had landed and Gary was with me. Then, we decided to stop for a quick bite to eat. He seemed happy to be eating real American food. As we ate, I filled him in as best I could about what had been happening with Brittany so he wouldn't be too shocked. I could tell by the look on his face it was worse than he expected. Because of his medical background, he understood what the possible outcomes were.

About an hour later, we arrived at the hospital. As we walked toward the building, we both looked at each other and took a deep breath. I smiled and gave him a pat on the shoulder. Neither of us said a word as we rode up in the elevator. All I could think about was how he would feel when he saw Brittany lying there. The door opened and I pointed to the right. As we started down the hall, several nurses walked toward us. They all raised their hands and started clapping softly for this soldier. He proudly kept on walking and smiled to the nurses as he passed them. I couldn't hold back my tears. As we walked by, several of them reached out and patted him on the back. I noticed some were wiping away tears because they knew why this soldier had been called home.

I pointed to the door of Brittany's room and waited for him to walk in first. Lori got up and came quickly to greet him and welcome him home. They hugged for a moment and then walked over to Brittany's bed. Her weak body kept her from hollering out in surprise like she normally would, but she had a big smile on her face. Gary moved the rail down on the bed and bent down to kiss her. Lori and I watched as her little arms reached up and around his neck. He had been gone so long, and she didn't want to let him go. He reached around her tiny body the best he could and just held her. There was no holding back the tears. As two nurses watched from the doorway, tears in their eyes told us they felt the emotion of that moment just as much as we did.

He sat on the edge of the bed, telling her how much he had missed her and how glad he was to be home. He was trying to hide his emotions, but the heartache he felt showed on his face. With all his medical training and experience, there was nothing he could do to help his own daughter. It was the same helpless feeling we all had to deal with. The two of them talked until Brittany's eyes finally closed. He sat for a few minutes gently rubbing her little hand.

Soon we heard footsteps behind us and turned to see who it was. Kat walked in wearing her usual smile. She had one of those smiles that always lifts you up.

She was happy to see that Gary had made it home. Lori introduced them and told him how she was helping. I sat in the chair by Brittany's bed and rubbed my hand over her arm while they talked. It was so hard to grasp all that was happening. There was so much, so fast. None of us had had time to just take a deep breath and relax.

After Gary and Kat got acquainted, Kat said, "Why don't you two take a breather and go somewhere quiet and talk. I'll stay here with Brittany."

Everything seemed under control, so I told Lori, "I think I'm going to get on home. Kat's here, and you and Gary have a lot to talk about. I'll call in the morning."

"Thank you, Mom," she said.

I hugged Lori and said, "Don't worry. Everything's going to be OK."

"Gary," I said, "it's good to have you home." I gave him a hug and a pat on the back.

Matt had Erik for the night, but I was going to pick him up in the morning and bring him to the hospital so he could see Brittany and spend some time with Lori and Gary. It would do them all a lot of good.

Across the street from the Children's Hospital was a home-away-from-home for family members of hospitalized children called the Ronald McDonald House. Since 1974, the non-profit organization that operated the Ronald McDonald House had been strengthening families during their most difficult and challenging times. The home

41

provides families with a place to sleep, shower, and wash clothes near the vicinity of their child. The hospital arranged for Lori and Gary to stay there so they would never be far away from Brittany. What a blessing that was.

Unexpected Complication

I needed to get caught up at work so I decided to go in for a few hours. My boss assured me that anytime I needed to leave I could. He could see how hard this was for me. The other people in the office were also supportive and always asked if I needed help with anything. I appreciated their kindness, but there really wasn't anything they could do that they weren't already doing.

It was hard to concentrate on work because I was constantly wondering what was happening at the hospital. After about an hour, I called Lori to see if there was any news.

"Hi, Sweetie, how's Brittany?"

"Well, she says she has a terrible pain in her stomach. I have no idea what it could be. I think something's wrong."

"Don't worry," I said. "Maybe it's because she isn't eating much. I'm going to take off and come on over. See you in a few."

As I drove, I looked up at the clouds in front of me. "God, are you there? Show me you are there. Please help our Brittany." I wanted to feel that closeness with God again.

I was always wondering if it was possible to heal another person if you prayed hard enough. I felt like I was praying harder than I ever had, but was more required than just prayer? What else do you need to do? What else can you do? It was hard to think about it all.

When I got to Brittany's room, Lori and Gary weren't there. I guessed they had gone to get a bite to eat. I walked over to Brittany and gave her a kiss on the cheek like I did each time I came to see her.

"Hi, Grandma," she said in a whisper. "My tummy hurts."

"Where does it hurt?" I asked. She put her hand on her lower abdomen. Right about then, a nurse came in. I wasn't shy about asking questions, so I mentioned it to the nurse. She said it would be helpful if we could get her up from her bed.

Brittany looked up at me and said, "Grammy, I have to go to the bathroom."

"Well, all right then. How about we get you out of this bed and stretch your legs. I bet it would feel good to walk a little, don't you think?" I could tell she really didn't want to, but she nodded her head yes. As I pulled the covers down and reached under her back to help her sit up, I quickly realized I would need help. It was a bit of work, but the nurse helped, and we got her up. It did my heart good just to see her feet touching the floor and taking steps. She kept her hand on her stomach as she walked bent over. I could see she was in pain, but she was trying.

I held on as we took one tiny step at a time. She walked slowly, but she did her best to keep moving. Again, she said her tummy hurt. I told her walking might make it better, but the pain in her eyes and voice made me think this wasn't a good idea. It was more of a struggle than I thought it would be. She was so weak, but we made it to the bathroom and back.

"You did so well," I told her. "Did it feel good to walk a little?"

"No, it still hurts," she answered.

"Well, let's get you comfortable, and I'll see if the nurse can give you something so it won't hurt."

As the nurse helped me get her back in bed, I told her I thought there was a problem with Brittany's stomach. She listed all the various things that could be causing it, as if it were normal under the circumstances. I insisted someone look at it anyway, and she agreed to inform the doctor. Later that day, we were told that they were going to X-ray her stomach to see what they could find.

It seemed they were taking her for some kind of test every day. By now, it wasn't uncommon for me to arrive and find Brittany not in her room. We were beginning to lose track of which test results we were waiting to hear about. Things were getting more and more confusing and jumbled up. I saw and felt the toll it was taking on my daughter and her husband. It was hard to think clearly and difficult to understand what was happening because there never seemed to be a resolution to anything.

When I arrived the next day, my daughter's face told me immediately that she had more bad news. I gave her a long hug and asked what was going on. Her head hung down in silence as we walked out into the hallway.

She took a deep breath and said in a shaky voice, "They found the reason Brittany's stomach was hurting so much. Somehow she has contracted a fungus called mucormycosis."

"What the heck is that?" I asked.

"Well, the doctor said it is a fungus that eats away at the body, just like the cancer. It attacks people with a low immune system, which she has. They aren't able to treat both the leukemia and the fungus at the same time, so they're going to have to stop the chemo to treat the fungus, and go back and forth. They have to treat one for a couple days and then the other."

"You're kidding." I said, "This is too much for a tiny, little person." I couldn't hold back the tears this time. "How can this be happening? I leaned my head back against the wall and wiped away the tears. I told Lori to go back in the room and I would be there in a minute. How would Brittany make it through something this extreme? She was so small and fragile. It was too much! There were no words to explain my feeling of helplessness.

I saw a doctor walk into the room, so I followed. I prayed he brought good news. He reached over and touched my daughter's shoulder as he got ready to speak. Gary quickly got up and came over. The three of us stood there, waiting to hear what he was going to say.

"There's a new drug that's being tested for this fungus and we're going to call Washington to see if they will release it so we can see if it will help Brittany."

I squeezed my daughter's hand, smiled, and said to the doctor, "Surely they will release it. No one would let a little child suffer if there was a chance to help them. Maybe she would be the one to save many lives in the future."

With a somewhat assuring voice he said, "We should hear from them tomorrow." He walked to Brittany's bed and smiled at her. As he felt her head for fever, he asked, "How is this pretty little gal doing?" She looked up, but didn't answer.

No wonder she's so exhausted all the time, I thought. Two diseases are eating away at her little body, but finally we had heard words that gave us some hope. Every minute her little body was suffering, and it was a relief to grab onto a fresh reason for optimism.

After the doctor left, Lori and Gary told Brittany what the doctor had told them about the new medicine. Her big brown eyes looked at them, but she still had no words. I went over and gave her a kiss on the cheek and said, "Sweetie Pie. Don't you worry; we're going to get you feeling better."

"Hey, where's your teddy bear?" I asked as I looked around. "I bet he wants to snuggle with you tonight. Ah ha, there he is. Let's put him right here where you can hold him so he doesn't fall out of bed." As I tucked it under her arm I said, "Sleep tight and don't let the bed bugs bite. I'm going now, but I'll see you in the morning."

Her sweet voice whispered, "OK, Grammy."

I felt it was all right to leave because I knew Barbara, Kat, or Dawn would be showing up soon. It was easier for them to do what they did when there weren't so many people watching. The three of them were continuing to visit every day. Because of their work schedules, they usually came in the evenings after I had left, so Lori and Gary saw them the most. Not one day went by without one or two of them showing up. Every day when I arrived, I asked Lori who came by, what they did, and what she thought about it. She always felt better after they had been there, but I was never sure if progress was being made.

I picked Erik up from the neighbor's house on my way home that night. He was such a happy little kid. I got the warmest feeling when he ran up and threw his little arms around my neck. He was still small enough that I could pick him up and give him a kiss, and that's what I did.

One of my favorite things to do with the kids was nibble on their neck and say, "Give me some sugar." They would laugh and squirm to get away, but they loved it.

When we got home, I got Erik ready for bed and climbed in beside him to read a story. We were both propped up against the headboard. He looked at me with his little hands palms up, about shoulder height, and said, "Where is Brittany?" I pulled him close and hugged him as I told him she was still at the hospital, but would be home soon. He slid out of bed and ran toward her room.

"Where are you going, Erik?" I asked.

He didn't say anything, but in a minute, he was back with one of Brittany's stuffed animals. He climbed back into bed and snuggled a little stuffed dog under his chin and waited for me to start reading. Usually, he never made it all the way through a story before nodding off.

As I lay in bed that night, I looked up through my ceiling to heaven and said a little prayer.

> *"Dear Lord, make them say yes to this new medicine. Please wrap Your arms around Lori and Gary and all the people in the hospital that work so hard to help these little children. Thank you for making doctors and nurses. I know there are lessons for us to learn, but right now, I can't think about that part. I will soon, I promise. Please give Brittany the strength to keep fighting."*

Driving to the hospital the next day, all I could think about was this new medicine and whether it would work. I knew with cancer, if you catch it early, you have a better chance of surviving, but I didn't know anything about this fungus. I tried to stay positive and was glad there was something new to try.

As I drove, I looked up, hoping to see another sign from God. There wasn't a fan of sunbeams like before; there were just clusters of clouds scattered about, leaving openings of blue sky. My eyes searched the sky as I prayed, "Anything, God, give me something, anything." I wanted desperately to feel His protection again.

Then I saw one single ray of light coming through a small hole in a cloud that pointed directly to the hospital. If you've watched clouds, you know that within seconds they can move and everything you see will look different, but for the next fifteen minutes, those clouds didn't move an inch. It was as if they were painted on the sky. The closer I got to the hospital, the brighter the light seemed as it streamed directly to the rooftop of the hospital. As I focused on that light, I felt we would hear good news.

When I arrived, Lori and Gary were sitting on Brittany's bed talking to her. I was thrilled to see that everyone was smiling.

"Hey, what's going on?" I asked in a cheerful voice.

My daughter stood up and said, "We have some good news, Mom. Washington has approved the new medicine and they are sending it overnight. It should be here tomorrow, and they'll start her on it right away."

I wanted to jump up and down like a little kid. For the first time in a long time, everyone was smiling. We even got a little bit of a smile out of Brittany. I was filled in on what the doctor had explained regarding how this drug was expected to work. It sounded promising. I took a giant breath and hugged them both. Everyone was in a good mood. I felt sure now that we would be going home within a week or so.

I sat down by Brittany and asked, "So, what have you guys been doing today?" Brittany held up the picture she had been coloring. It was a princess and a unicorn in a garden. "Oh my, you have made her look beautiful!" She smiled and put it back on her lap to finish. Just then, a woman brought in a tray with her lunch. There wasn't much there, just some soup and jello.

"Oh look, Brittany. You have jello. Yum, that looks good." She glanced at the jello, then back to her picture, and continued to color.

"I don't want any right now," she said.

"How about you take just a couple bites? I'll help you."

She was quick to answer back, "No, my tummy doesn't want any." I looked at Lori and Gary to see their response. They just shrugged and gave me an "it's OK" look.

Lori pulled me aside and told me, "She hardly eats anything, Mom. Eating makes her feel sick."

With a worried voice I said, "But she's withering away, Lori."

"I know, Mom. We keep trying, but she just won't."

Again I wanted to hug Brittany or at least give her a comforting touch, but I couldn't. Because of the constant pain, Brittany was now being given frequent doses of morphine. After just a week of this, it had made her skin so sensitive that she would feel pain if you just rubbed her arm or held her hand. It broke our hearts to think touching her would hurt her. How could we not touch her? That's how we give comfort and love. I wasn't sure how to deal with that. The struggle to understand heightened at times like these.

Wanting to lighten things up, Gary bought a small foam baseball bat so she could bat away the doctors and nurses. She didn't have enough energy to hit hard, and, of course, she really didn't do it in a mean way. It was mainly something to help take her mind off how she was feeling. We had always been careful to explain why the doctors and nurses needed to do certain things so she would understand everyone was on her side trying to make her well.

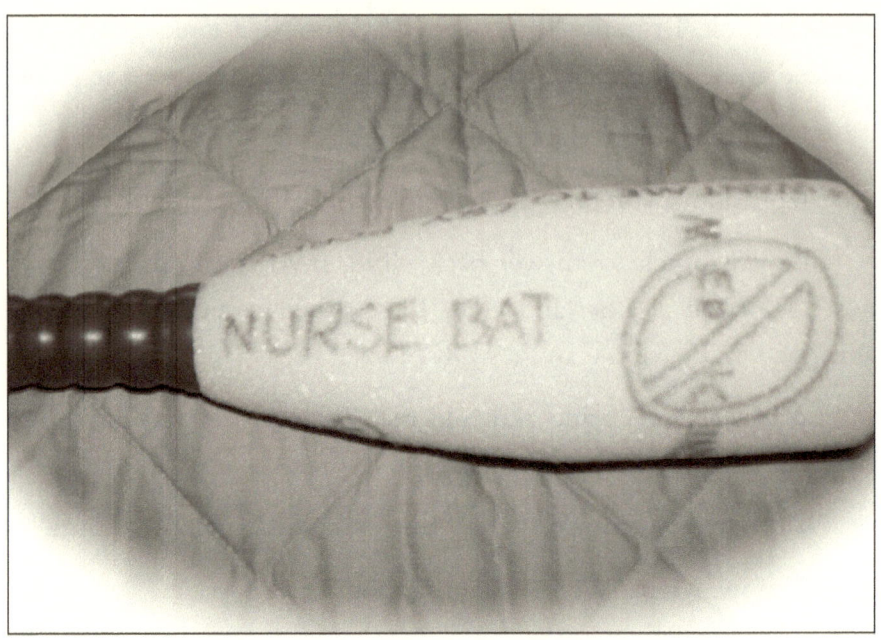

Together, Brittany and her dad had come up with things to write on the bat. On one side, he wrote "Nurse Bat." Then he wrote the word "Medicine" and added a circle with a line through it. It was fun to watch them get the bat all set up. They seemed to be having a good time.

"OK," Gary asked Brittany. "What else should we write?"

"Umm," she said with a slight chuckle, "you can write 'Get Away'."

"OK," he said and wrote it on the bat. Next he drew a hand and wrote "STOP" underneath it. When they had filled in almost every spot, she was ready for action. There she lay, with bat in hand, waiting for the next nurse. The nurses and doctors were good sports and played along. They would creep up on her in a playful way and then duck from the bat before letting her bop them on the head.

Her dad told her there were good guys and bad guys in her body, and right now, the bad guys were winning. He told her that if she took her medicine, the good guys could fight harder and win. He was the only one who could get her to take pills. We had been careful to explain to her that her sickness would make her lose her hair. We weren't sure how she would take that, but to our surprise, it didn't seem to bother her. Sometimes it seemed she understood more about what was happening than we did. She never cried or even seemed afraid.

We were expecting Lori's Aunt Kathy and her grandmother to be arriving soon from Utah. Brittany knew they were coming and was excited to see them. They had always played a big part in the lives of my kids and continued to do so with Brittany and Erik and the other grandchildren. About an hour later as Lori, Gary, and I sat in the room chatting, I noticed them in the hall outside the door. This would be the first time they saw Brittany looking so pale and lying so still. I knew they would be shocked and would have a hard time containing their feelings.

I walked over to greet them. "I'm so glad you're here," I said, and gave them both a hug. I could see they were fighting back tears. I felt my throat burning as I fought to hold back my own tears. Lori and Gary came over and hugged them both before they went over to Brittany's bed.

As they walked toward the bed, I watched their faces. I knew this would be hard for them. They were heart sick, but did a good job of not showing Brittany. Her eyes lit up when she saw them. Kathy leaned over and gave her a kiss. "We had heard so much about California, we just had to come and visit. It's freezing in Utah right now. We have to get you better so you can take us to the beach!"

"I want to go home," Brittany told her. "I want to go to school. My friends drew me some pictures, see?" She pointed to the wall.

Kathy replied, "You sure have a lot of friends. Look at all those pictures."

Lori's grandmother, Melba, reached over to squeeze her hand and was surprised when Brittany pulled away.

"It hurts when you do that," Brittany told her. I could see that Melba was crushed. No one had thought ahead of time to warn her. I felt so bad. I knew she wanted to give Brittany a big hug like she always did. This was one of the hardest things for all of us to adjust to. We could only touch her if we did so very gently.

Lori, Gary, and I backed away for a while and let Kathy and Melba talk as long as Brittany was able. Soon it was time for her shot of morphine. They watched as the nurse put it in the tube that came out of her chest. I could tell by the expressions on their faces that they were wondering about the tube, so Lori explained what it was. We had kept them updated by phone, but when everything is right in front of you, it's a different story. The heartbreak that comes is devastating. Soon Brittany's eyes closed for the night.

We all sat and talked for a while about what the future might hold. Keeping faith and hope alive was our biggest challenge. No one was sure how long Brittany would be in the hospital, so Kathy suggested they take Erik back to Utah with them until Brittany was better. Considering the circumstances, Lori and Gary decided it would be a good idea. Erik knew them well, so it would be an easy transition for him. They weren't leaving for a few days, so Lori and Gary would be able to spend some time with him before he left.

It was getting late, so Kathy and Melba decided to leave and take Erik back to the house with them for the night. As they were getting ready to leave, Barbara came in. Lori introduced Barbara and explained what she was doing to help Brittany. What they heard was new to them, but they did their best to understand. They graciously thanked Barbara for taking time to work with Brittany. Everything going on was new and unexpected. We knew the hospital staff had things under control, but we still felt helpless and unprepared. Kathy, Melba, and I left Barbara there to do her work with Brittany, bringing her, we hoped, one step closer to going home.

Sometimes I didn't know if Brittany was sleeping or just too tired to keep her eyes open. Just a couple weeks ago she had been running, playing, and dancing around the house.

I remembered how cute she had looked all dressed up in her pink ballerina outfit. I loved taking pictures of the kids, and one day Brittany and I had decided to do a ballerina photo shoot. We shuffled through the drawers looking for all the pieces. We needed the leotard, the tights, the tutu, and a flower for her hair. Once she was all dressed, I combed and fluffed her hair and we were ready to go. It was so much fun. If I had had a tutu for myself, I would have put it on, too. I showed Brittany the poses I remembered from my ballerina days and started snapping pictures as she did each one. After a few pictures, we danced around the room as if we were performing on stage.

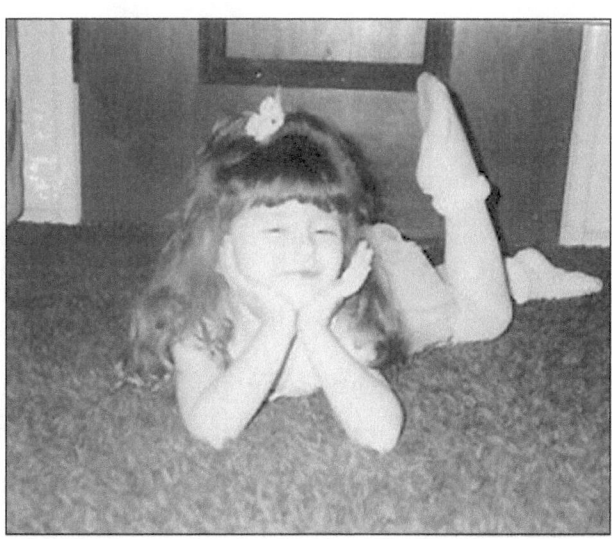

There were days when the hospital room became filled with new hope. On Sunday, when the doctor came in for his morning visit, he was smiling. It was hard to tell what his smile meant because all the staff smiled a lot. We had been told the day before that the new medicine was being sent overnight, so we hoped he was smiling because it had arrived.

"I have some good news for you," he said. "The new drug arrived this morning and we are ready to begin treatment. Since this is still in the testing phase, I can't promise anything, but there is a good chance we will be successful." That was truly music to our ears. He went on to explain how it worked and what they hoped would happen.

"See," I said, as I hugged my daughter and her husband. "Things are looking up. It's going to be OK. Keep believing that it's going to be OK."

About fifteen minutes later, a nurse came in with the medicine. Brittany picked up her bat and gave it a little swing. The nurse played along with her and ducked from the bat as she smiled.

"Hey, Brittany," she said. "We have a new medicine for you. Soon you will be running and playing. I don't even have to stick you with a needle." Lori and Gary stood on the other side of the bed while she put the medicine in the tube in her chest.

The nurse smiled at Brittany and said, "There, see, that didn't hurt at all." She smiled at Lori and Gary and held up her hand with crossed fingers. Everyone was hoping for the best.

Here we were again, waiting for good news . . . waiting to see if our little Brittany would get well and live a normal life again. We wanted to hear her laugh and see her run and play again.

A Visit From The LA Times

The next afternoon, Kathy and Melba came for a visit and brought Erik. When he saw his mom and dad, he ran to them. Lori reached down and scooped him up. His arms wrapped around her neck as she held him in her arms and pressed her head against his cheek. They rocked slowly back and forth while his arms stayed wrapped around her. She lifted her head and kissed his face and walked to Brittany's bed. He wanted to climb in the bed with her, but of course, we couldn't let him.

Lori leaned in closer so their little fingers could touch for a brief moment. Brittany knew he liked her teddy bear so she held it up to show him. As he giggled and reached for it, she moved it closer to him so he could take it and hold it for a minute. He kissed the bear's face, laughed, and hugged it tight under his chin. Then he giggled again and leaned forward to give it back to Brittany. He was just a little tike and full of energy, so it was hard for him to be still for too long. Gary noticed he was getting restless and took him out in the hall where he could walk around a bit.

It was great to see Gary and Erik together. Erik was a little Gary Jr. Even at his young age, they looked so much alike and shared a lot of the same characteristics. It was fun watching them interact. Gary was so happy to be back with his family.

Lori told me that a reporter from the *LA Times* would soon be coming by for an interview. Someone at the Red Cross had told them about Gary being brought home to be with his daughter, and now they wanted to do a story for the Sunday paper. They had called Lori and Gary three times to get permission and were told NO the first two times because it seemed awkward and didn't feel right. The third time, they finally said yes.

Around two o'clock, I noticed a woman dressed in a suit clutching a notepad, standing at the doorway talking to a nurse. After a few minutes, the nurse pointed our way. The woman walked in the room and came over to my daughter and her husband. She was the *LA Times* reporter.

Kathy and Melba took Erik out of the room so we could talk with the reporter. For the next thirty minutes or so, the woman talked to Lori, Gary, and me about Brittany, her condition, and how Gary had been brought home from the Gulf War to be with her.

For some reason, listening to everything was making me angry. It felt like we were talking about Brittany as if she only had days to live. I wanted to scream out, "She's going to be fine, you know!" I didn't feel like doing this interview anymore. I turned away and went over to Brittany. She gave me a little smile and I smiled back. I touched her cheek to see if she felt warm.

"You know what, Brittany," I said. "Tomorrow I'll bring Dollie Wollie and we can comb her hair and paint her fingernails." Her eyes popped open, and she seem excited about seeing her favorite doll.

"OK," she answered. A burst of happiness swept over me. Seeing her feel even a tiny bit of excitement was always uplifting.

After the interview, the reporter asked if she could photograph Brittany with her mom and dad sitting with her on the bed. Again, they wondered if they should say yes. Something about it didn't feel right. It wasn't my decision, so I went across the room and stood quietly in the corner. My heart felt heavy and sad. I looked at Brittany lying there and wondered what she must be thinking.

With the help of a nurse, Lori and Gary managed to exchange Brittany's hospital gown for a dress. Then they each went to one side of her bed and sat beside her. Just then, Erik came running into the room, so Gary picked him up and put him on his lap so that he could be in the photograph. I don't think any of us realized how tiring all this was for Brittany. Her head rolled a little to one side as she stared ahead. It was heartbreaking to watch. Where was that cute little girl full of life . . . the one who always danced around the house and made us smile? Again, I wanted to pick her up, take her home, and pretend none of this had happened.

As the photos were snapped, her expression didn't change. She didn't seem to care what was going on. She held her little white lamb loosely as if it didn't matter if it was even there.

The reporter told us the story would be printed in the Sunday paper. I hoped she didn't plan to call every day to see if there was something new to write about. I had a hard time dealing with this whole idea. This was private. Why would strangers want to read about it? There was nothing they could do. To them, it was just a sad story they would soon forget.

There was another girl about Brittany's age in the bed right across from her. When the interview and pictures were over, I heard her ask her mom, "Why don't they take pictures of me?" I didn't hear her mother's answer, but I couldn't help but wonder what goes on in the minds of these kids while they are going through this. I'm sure they are scared and don't understand what's happening to them or how serious it could be.

Kathy and Melba spent the next half hour talking with Brittany before taking Erik back to the house. They gave Brittany kisses and said they would see her tomorrow. As we walked out to the hallway, everyone's eyes got teary. We all were experiencing the same feeling of helplessness. There seemed to be nothing we could do to make any of it better.

The Rose

The constant wondering about what would happen wore us all down. Kathy, Melba, and Erik had left for the day, and I knew Lori and Gary needed a break.

"You two go get some lunch and relax a bit." I said. "I'll sit with Brittany."

They took off, and I sat down beside the bed. Brittany's eyes looked heavy, and I thought reading would help her fall asleep. I picked up *The Little Mermaid* and began reading. Within five minutes, her eyes closed. I knew she would sleep for a while, so I decided to go out to the garden we had visited on our wagon ride.

I took the elevator down to the first floor and found my way to the garden. The sun was still shining and the scent of flowers lured me over to a little white bench. While sitting there, I noticed something out of the corner of my eye and turned to see what it was. There beside me, almost close enough to touch was a beautiful rose bush filled with fully bloomed roses. They were . . . pink! A mixture of happiness and sadness came over me. I leaned forward to breathe in their fragrance. No wonder Brittany cherished them so much. They smelled lovely, were beautiful to look at, and were the perfect color for a sweet little girl.

I smiled to myself as I pulled my car keys out of my purse. Surely a key would be sharp enough to cut a stem. I found the prettiest rose and then looked around to see if anyone was watching. I pressed the key against the stem and snap! Ah ha! Perfect. I would take this back for my sweet Brittany.

I stared at the rose bush and realized this was a moment to cherish. The garden had many warm and peaceful places to sit, but for some reason I had sat down by a pink rose without even realizing it. God has a way of helping us find what we need. Perhaps I had seen this rose bush the last time we were there, but didn't pay attention, so it called me back to let me know I had a place to come and sit. I felt at peace there, so I sat for a while, enjoying the moment.

It's interesting how we choose objects, sounds, or colors to help us create moments we will never forget. Some people love butterflies or hummingbirds. Some collect coins or shark teeth along the beach. Some will never miss the county fair. Do you ever wonder why certain people decide what they do? It doesn't really matter what we do; what matters is why we do it. Each of us has our own reasons.

While walking back to Brittany's room, I remembered a small quilt she had with pink roses on it. The quilt was her favorite, of course. I stopped at the nurses' station and got a paper and pen so I could write myself a note. I wrote: "Bring pink rose quilt and Dolly Wollie." I was sure that having the quilt on her bed would make her feel at home.

One of the nurses noticed I was holding the freshly cut pink rose. She smiled and said, "That's a beautiful rose. Would you like something to put it in?"

I smiled a guilty kind of smile and said, "Yes, that would be nice. Thank you." I'm sure she knew I had cut it from the garden, but just like the roses Brittany had picked not so long ago for my daughter and me, it was picked for the joy of giving.

When I got back to the room, Brittany was sleeping, and Lori and Gary were talking. I held up the rose and smiled as I placed it on the table by Brittany's bed. They smiled back, knowing Brittany would love waking to see her favorite flower.

Lori said Barbara would be coming by soon and Kat was planning to come later that evening.

"OK, then," I said, "You are in good hands. I think I'll mosey on home." We shared our usual hugs and I gathered up my things.

"Thanks, Mom," Lori said. "I'll see you tomorrow."

"Good night, Sweetie. You and Gary try to get some rest. They will look after Brittany. You need to sleep."

As I headed toward the elevator, I tried not to look in the rooms. I did listen, though. Some of the rooms were completely silent. From others, I heard children laughing and playing games. The nurses told me that some of the kids come for a few days once a month for treatment and were doing well. It was good to know that some defeat this terrible disease and go on to lead normal lives.

As I passed the last nurses' station, I noticed a small calendar propped up on the counter about the size of a three-by-five index card. On the space to the right of the calendar was a small pink rose. Seeing it there gave me butterflies in my stomach. I know pink roses are not uncommon. You see them on many items in many places, but because Brittany loved them so much, I had always made it a big deal whenever I saw one.

As I drove home, I turned on the radio, hoping to hear something that would rest my mind. I took a deep breath and thought, "Dear God, what is this all about?" Why do people have to get sick, especially little children? Why do they have to suffer and be afraid? It seems so cruel. Why does there have to be so much heartache?

A song started to play on the radio and the first three beats caught my attention. I listened attentively until I recognized the song and the voice. It was Bette Midler, and the song was *The Rose*. I had heard the song many times, but this time, I listened intently. It was a beautiful message about how much of life you lose because you are afraid to love and live without fear. Yes, love can hurt, but it is also the greatest gift we have to give to others. I think we use fear as a way to protect ourselves from getting hurt, but in the process, we miss some of the most beautiful and heartwarming experiences life can give us. We come into this world with a loving heart and we leave with a loving heart. Love is the one thing no one can take from us. The song is short but powerful, and so full of meaning if you stop and listen. The message will remain in my mind and heart forever. For me, this was now Brittany's song. It goes like this:

The Rose

By Amanda McBroom

Some say love, it is a river that drowns the tender reed.

Some say love, it is a razor that leads your soul to bleed.

Some say love, it is a hunger, an endless aching need.

I say love; it is a flower and you its only seed.

It's the heart, afraid of breaking that never learns to dance.

It's the dream afraid of waking that never takes the chance.

It's the one who won't be taken who cannot seem to give.

And the soul afraid of dying that never learns to live.

When the night has been too lonely and the road has been too long,

And you think that love is only for the lucky and the strong.

Just remember in the winter, far beneath the bitter snow.

Lies the seed that with the sun's love, in the spring becomes the rose.

I wondered if Brittany's sickness was about teaching us this message. Could this be the answer to why all this is happening? Part of me felt relieved to think I had found the purpose of this experience, but another part of me was terrified. Was her life's purpose to be a teacher, to teach us this lesson and then leave us? Oh God, please don't take her!

For the rest of the evening, I attempted to make sense of the day's events. My heart said one thing, and my mind said another. They would agree, then disagree, then agree again. Maybe I was trying too hard to figure it all out. Was this where faith comes in? Should we just have more faith and stop trying to figure it out?

One thing I was becoming more sure of was that I was being sent divine inspiration, bit-by-bit. Roses, especially pink ones, had a special importance to us, and that day they had made their presence known as messengers from God. "Stop and smell the roses" was living up to its message. Although I was still confused and afraid, these events were making me stronger. I realized that more than ever, I needed to pay close attention to everything that went on around me. These experiences were the first of many that would use the rose to teach me life lessons.

Chapter Two

Hope Holds Us Together

A New Day

On the previous day, the hospital staff had moved Brittany to her own room so we could have more privacy with fewer disturbances. The room had pale yellow walls that made it cozy and warm. Brittany seemed to feel more comfortable there. It was also easier for Barbara, Kat, and Dawn to do their work without others watching and wondering what they were doing.

I had followed everyone to the new room and saw in the corner a soft and comfortable looking chair, so I went over and sat down. In a daze, I watched the nurses get Brittany settled and comfortable. My mind reeled as I started thinking of the events that had brought us to where we were. In just a few weeks, so much had happened. One day had started with two lovely pink roses and had ended with Brittany becoming desperately ill. The Red Cross had brought her father home from war. Three wonderful women had appeared in our lives to help us get through one of the toughest experiences anyone ever faces. God had sent a vision of sunbeams to comfort me. A teacher who none of us knew had her class send Get Well cards. The song *The Rose* had started playing on the radio at just the right time. Roses were appearing and making their connection known. Washington had released a new medicine, and Brittany had been given a private room where we could sit together and work it all out.

Today, I was headed to Brittany's new room carrying Dollie Wollie and the pink rose quilt. No one had called during the night, which meant nothing had changed for the worse.

"What's going on today?" I asked Gary as I walked in.

"Well," he answered, "the new medicine for the fungus doesn't seem to make her as sick as the chemo treatment, so she feels a little better today."

"Do they know yet if it's working?" I asked.

"Not yet," he answered. "The doctor said in a couple days they'll run more tests to see if there is any improvement."

"Good," I said. "We just have to be patient. They're doing all they can and this is a good hospital, so don't worry. It's going to be OK."

Brittany was awake and seemed more alert, so I decided that meant the new medicine was working. With a big smile I said, "Guess what I have?" I reached in my bag and pulled out Dollie Wollie. She was so happy to see her doll. When I handed it to her, she pulled it to her chest and hugged it.

"I brought some extra clothes for her, too. What should we dress her in today?" I asked.

"She likes the blue dress with the white ruffle," she answered. She watched as I put the blue dress on the doll.

"Here's a brush. Do you want to brush her hair?" I asked.

"OK," she answered in a tiny voice. I handed her the brush and she began brushing Dollie Wollie's hair.

"Now, when you get done making her pretty, we can paint her fingernails."

"All right," she answered.

When she was done brushing Dolly Wollie's hair, I got out the fingernail polish. "Shall we paint her nails first and then yours?"

"OK," she said, so I started painting the doll's fingernails. I painted one finger and showed Brittany.

"What do you think of this color? It's pink just like a pink rose."

"It looks pretty," she replied in a quiet voice. She wasn't as enthusiastic as normal, but it seemed to entertaining her somewhat.

All of a sudden I heard her say, "Grandma, my eyes are burning!" Right away, I knew it was the nail polish. I quickly put the lid on the bottle and moved the doll to the chair.

"Oh, Sweetie, I'm so sorry." I ran to the sink and got a cold washcloth to put over her eyes. Luckily, within seconds her eyes stopped burning. I felt horrible. Why didn't I realize that might happen?

Trying to change the subject I said, "Guess what else I brought?"

"What, Grandma? What did you bring?" I reached in my bag again and pulled out her quilt with the pink roses. "I thought you would like to have your favorite quilt." She smiled as I handed it to her. I laid it on the bed and pulled it up around her chest. She kept looking at it and rubbing her fingers over the little roses.

"Thank you, Grandma," she said.

I reached into my purse and got out a tiny pink bear we often played with. Brittany had named her Rose. It was a little pink finger puppet that fit perfectly on my index finger. I would be the voice of Rose, and we would have fun little conversations. This was how we passed the time.

Around two o'clock, Kathy and Melba came for a visit. They would be returning to Utah the next day with Erik, so this was their last day to be with Brittany. The sadness in their faces made it clear that they wondered if this was the last time they would see her. I suggested Lori and Gary go to the house and spend some time with Erik that evening. Things were changing, and we all were having a hard time accepting how it would affect each of us.

After Kathy and Melba left, I stayed with Brittany until Kat came. When she arrived, I was the only one in the room, and I was glad for the chance to get to know her better. She was kind, patient, and smiled a lot, and the calming effect she radiated was amazing. She spent the next half hour explaining to me how the healing work she did was for all of us, not just Brittany. She spoke softly and always looked right into my eyes. I tried to pay attention to all she was saying, but I wanted to stop her and say, "But, aren't you here to heal Brittany?" I didn't want her to spend time healing us, because Brittany needed all her attention right now. Even though she explained her work to me, I didn't have a clear understanding of what to expect. I did my best to take in what she said and have faith that more understanding would come. Brittany was sleeping and I knew Kat wanted to do her work, so I thanked her for spending time with me and said good night.

SOMETHING TO BELIEVE IN

The next afternoon, Barbara came by for a visit. She brought a few new Hemi-Sync tapes for us to try. The idea of how they worked was fascinating. I wondered how someone figured it all out. Although we didn't completely understand what the outcome was supposed to be, we were willing to try anything that made sense. Brittany had taken to all three of these women almost instantly. Lori and Gary were amazed at how well they all worked together. For the next little while, we let Barbara and Brittany enjoy some conversation.

I had the feeling there was also some kind of message for us in the healing work these three were doing, but I couldn't put my finger on what it was. It was all still confusing. Were these "healers" going to heal Brittany or not? Why didn't she seem to be getting better? Does the amount of faith we have make a difference to her living or dying? I still didn't completely understand how to feel about any of it.

Gary took the opportunity of Barbara's visit to go out and take care of a few things. He had to find some kind of transportation, so he needed to look for a car. He also needed to buy some clothes. The only clothes he had were tucked away in his small backpack. I felt so bad for him. He never complained, but I knew there was so much going through his head. He had left the battlefield of war only to come home to a different kind of battle.

Once Barbara got Brittany set up for listening to the tapes, she told us about a man named Sai Baba who lived in India and who was considered a saint by his many followers. They thought of him in the same way some people think of Jesus. It was believed that he was able to send healing powers anywhere in the world and was able to manifest material objects at times. I wasn't sure about that, but tried to remain open minded. Lori jumped at the chance to learn more about him. Barbara told us there was a Sai Baba Center nearby that we could visit if we were interested and offered to sit with Brittany if we wanted to go. Gary was running his errands, so Lori and I decided to make a visit to the center, which was only about a ten-minute drive away.

The front area was set up like a small store with pictures, books, and other holy items from India. Lori took a book from the shelf and began reading about Sai Baba. One page showed a small medallion about the size of a dime with his face on one side and a holy symbol on the other. It was supposed to bring healing powers to the wearer.

She brought the book over to me and said, "Look, Mom, let's look for one of these. I could put it on a chain and hang it over Brittany's bed."

"OK," I said, "let's look." I wasn't sure if it would help, but I also wasn't sure that it wouldn't. We looked everywhere in the store, but couldn't find the medallion.

"Maybe they don't have any," I suggested.

"Well," Lori answered, "they should. I see they have some of the other things that were in the book. The book says this medallion can send healing energy. Let's keep looking."

"OK," I said. As we walked around, we noticed a room with red velvet curtains on every wall. The furniture was also velvet and different holy items were leaning against the walls. It was a place to sit and meditate, so we did just that. It's strange where your mind goes in situations like this. We were really reaching out and doing our best to have faith in everyone and everything without judgment.

We sat without speaking, hoping to feel something extraordinary come over us. We were desperate to feel a spiritual power reveal a promising message. We sat on the floor with our eyes closed and each said our own silent prayer. We even did some deep breathing to open our minds and hearts to heaven. Maybe we were trying too hard, because nothing extraordinary happened. We did leave the room feeling much calmer, though, so maybe that's all that moment was meant to be.

Lori still wanted to look for the medallion, so off we went on our hunt. She wasn't going to give up easily. Her mind was set on finding it.

She noticed an open door at the back of the room. "Let's go see what's in there," she said. As we walked toward the door, I looked behind me to see if anyone was going to stop us. No one was watching, so we went in. Cabinets stood against every wall. One tall cabinet caught Lori's attention because it had about twenty small drawers in it. She figured a small item would be in a small drawer, so she began opening the drawers one by one.

After looking through several drawers, I heard her say, "Mom, look! Here it is! There's only one left. Can you believe that?" She was so happy to find it. Only one left, and she found it in a room that wasn't open to the public. Did something draw us to that room so she would find the medallion?

I didn't know what to say. Shock and excitement bounced back and forth inside my head. I wanted to believe a heavenly power intervened and put it there for her to find.

We went back into the front of the store to buy the medallion, along with some pictures of Sai Baba and a book about his life. Why not learn more, I thought. For all we knew, this could be the one thing that would change it all for the better. You have to believe. If you don't, you have nothing.

Lori laid her items on the counter so the clerk could calculate the price. When the woman picked up the medallion, her eyes got big. Lori and I stared at her, wondering why she looked so startled.

She asked Lori, "Where did you get this?" Lori told her and said how happy she was to get the last one.

The woman replied. "I can't believe it. These are popular and hard to come by. We have never been able to get them for our store. I've been here for five years and this is the first one I've seen."

Chills ran through us as we stared at each other, wondering how the medallion got there. Was it manifested specifically for Lori?

Lori took a deep breath and asked the woman if she had a chain to put the medallion on. She quickly said no. Since she was so quick to answer, we guessed they never had those, either.

As we were gathering up our things, I could hear the woman opening and closing the sliding glass doors to a cupboard behind her. Just as we were ready to walk out the door, we heard her say,

"Oh, wait. Here's one. Will this work?" We walked back and took a look.

"Perfect," Lori answered. "Yes, this would be perfect." Again, we looked at each other in amazement. What were we to make of this? On our way back to the hospital, we talked about what we thought of the experience and how much believing in things made a difference and helped us to carry on. At that particular time, hope was all we had, and we weren't going to give it up.

I thought, was it a coincidence? Or, were we being sent an experience that would stimulate our insight? How did we get this medallion they said they never bought? Did this holy man in India manifest it for us? After all, that's what they said he could do. Would we ever know for sure? Did we need to know for sure? There was a lesson somewhere that would be sorted out in time. At that moment, I felt it was there for Lori. It lifted her spirits and gave her a new reason to believe. We were always grateful for moments that we interpreted as divine influence.

When we arrived back at the hospital, Brittany wasn't in her bed. A moment of panic always seized us when we didn't see her there, but since Gary and Barbara were sitting calmly across the room, we figured Brittany had been taken for more tests. Lori asked Gary where Brittany was.

He said, "They took her to do a biopsy on her stomach and see if the new medicine is working." We were relieved, and hoped we would hear something positive soon.

Lori showed Gary and Barbara the medallion and told them the story.

"You're kidding," Gary said. "I guess it was meant to be." His open-minded attitude was always a blessing. Being willing to consider new ideas helped us to survive the anxious moments we were constantly experiencing.

Finding the medallion seemed to wrap a little bubble of hope around us. The mood in the room was somewhat calmer, but there was still some nervous anticipation as to how Brittany would react to this new medicine.

Barbara smiled and said she was glad to hear we had such an uplifting experience at the center. The look on her face was not one of surprise. It was as if she knew this would happen. She was a firm believer in the spiritual realm and always brought us great comfort.

I sat in the corner thinking to myself. What does it take to feel connected to the spirit world and feel so sure of things like Barbara does? Are you born that way or can you learn? Some say we all have the ability to be spiritually connected to the world beyond and can develop it further if we make the effort to do so.

As we waited for Brittany to return, Lori put the medallion on the chain and hung it over her bed. She put the picture of Sai Baba on the wall where Brittany could see it. I watched quietly as Lori and Gary prepared this new spark of hope. In their hearts, they were hoping for a miracle. We all sat in silence for a few minutes as we digested the day's events.

Gary finally broke the silence by saying, "I found a car." We had completely forgotten he had gone looking for one.

"You did? Good." Lori replied. "What did you get?"

"It's an older VW van, but it seems to run OK." Something was always breaking down on the older cars we all drove, but Gary was mechanically inclined, so if anything went wrong, he could fix it.

As we were talking, a doctor came in. The doctors didn't usually stop by unless they had something to tell you, so we were eager to hear what was up.

"Well," he said, "it appears the drug is working. The fungus doesn't seem to be progressing. We just need to wait a little longer to make sure the existing diseased cells die."

"How long will that take?" Lori asked.

"We'll check again in a few days. We'll know for sure by then."

That news made our day! We thanked him and asked when Brittany would be returning.

"We sedated her, so she's in recovery right now. She'll be here within the next half hour, but will probably sleep. This would be a good time for you to get a bite to eat if you're hungry."

Barbara said Brittany had listened to the tapes for a good while that day and rested peacefully while doing so. When they took her for the biopsy, she showed no fear at all. Having all this help was unbelievable. It was hard to comprehend all that had happened, and how many people had come to help.

FROM DESERT TO DAUGHTER'S SIDE

The day had finally come for the article to be printed in the *LA Times*. We were so occupied with what was going on, we hadn't remembered to buy a paper. Around ten o'clock that morning, a nurse brought in the paper and asked if we had seen it. None of us had, so we were eager to see what had been written. She handed Lori the paper and we all huddled around. We stood in silence as we looked at the half-page picture of Lori, Gary, Erik, and Brittany sitting on the hospital bed. All I could think was, "Oh dear God, please don't let this be their last family portrait."

The headline read, "From Desert to Daughter's Side."

The subheading read, "The Army, moving with quickness and compassion, speeds a father from the front lines of Saudi Arabia to be with his 4-year-old daughter, just diagnosed with leukemia."

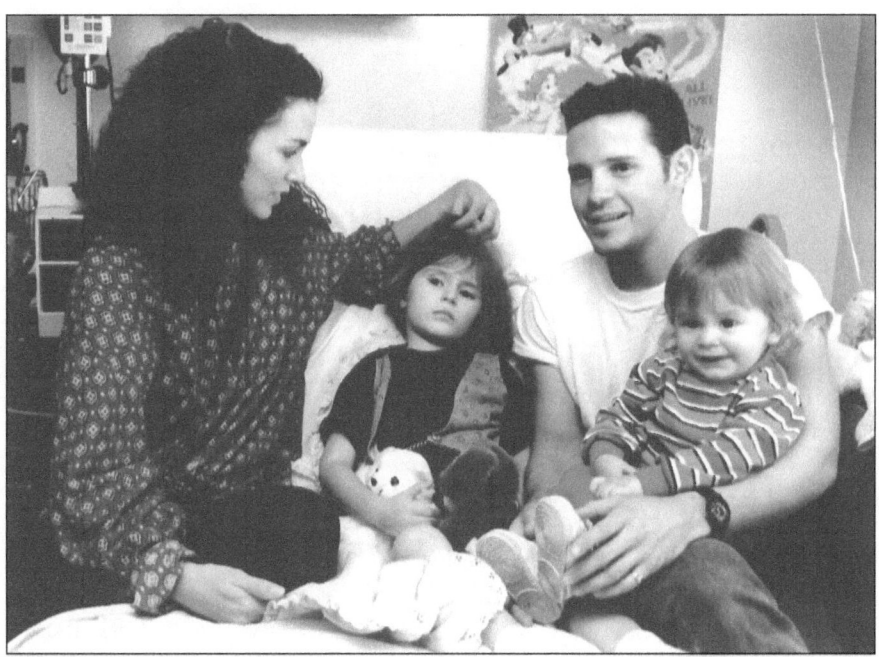

Trying to read the article aloud was much too emotional, so we each took turns reading it on our own. It was like something from a movie, so unreal.

The reporter had asked Brittany what she did when she first saw her dad. "I told him I missed him. I couldn't run to him because I was hooked up to that thing," she said, pointing to the bedside monitoring machine that tracked her vital signs.

I was the last to read the article and when done, set the paper on a table in the corner. No one knew what to say. At that point, it was only part of a story, with no ending. I think the same weird feeling came over each of us as we realized people we didn't even know would read the story on their train ride to work or as they sipped their morning coffee at home. They would feel sad for a while, but would soon forget as they got on with their day. I wasn't sure why we had agreed to do the interview in the first place. What good could come out of it?

THE BLUE BLITZ SOCCER TEAM

Dawn was there when I got to the hospital. She was like a warm blanket on a cold winter's night. Her calm voice made you feel better even if you didn't understand everything she was saying. Sometimes she did her healing work on Brittany, and other times, she sat and talked with us, which was also her healing power at work. She stayed for about an hour that day talking with us and doing some healing work on Brittany. Brittany was always quiet and calm when Dawn was there. Constantly, I wondered if that meant the healing was working or if she was just too tired to move. I hated the fact that I kept questioning the very things I wanted to have more faith in.

Later that afternoon, the nurse brought in a letter addressed to Brittany. It was from a girl in the neighboring city of Irvine named Kaley Pickett.

Here is what she wrote:

February 5, 1991

Dear Brittany,

You don't know me, but I know all about you. My name is Kaley Pickett and I am 9 years old and read an article in the Los Angeles Times newspaper about you on Sunday morning. I was so sad to hear that you weren't feeling well.

I am currently on the Irvine All Star Blue Blitz Soccer Team. We had our hardest game of this season yesterday. On the way to the game I said to my mom that I didn't think we could win and she said it wasn't that important when you think about what Brittany is going through. Then we said, "Let's win this game for Brittany." We also decided that if we did win, we would write you and tell you all about it. Well, we did win! The score was 5 to 1 and the last time we played that team, we had lost 3 to 1. You can imagine how excited we were and it is all because you are good luck to us. We also won our second game with a score of 5 to 0 and dedicated both games to you.

Today, the whole team got together and decided that not only would we write to you, but that each girl would pledge $1.00 for every goal the team scored for Blue Blitz for Brittany.

Brittany, you are an inspiration to our team. We know that sometimes things are hard, but that is when you have to try your hardest! You can never give up! Our team has such wonderful thoughts for you and we feel that you are good luck to us. Since we won our toughest battle, we know you will too!

We love you and you are in our thoughts and prayers everyday! All of us hope that we will get a chance to meet you soon!

Love,

Kaley Pickett

BBB (Blue Blitz for Brittany)

We were all overtaken with tears, amazed that this young girl was so moved by our story that she took action on the feelings in her heart. It was incredible to see how the events in your life branch out to other people.

Since there was a phone number on the letter, Lori asked me if I would call and thank her. When I called, I reached their answering machine, so I left a message saying who I was and that we had received the letter from Kaley. I told her how grateful we were and that I would call again later when I got home.

When I got home that evening, I had a message from a woman named Nancy. I didn't know anyone named Nancy, but since the caller had a sweet and warm voice, I called back. When a woman answered, I introduced myself and said I had gotten a message from Nancy. She told me she was Nancy, Kaley's mother. I told her we had received Kaleys' letter and were greatly moved by it. She began by telling me how after reading the story about Brittany, Kaley wanted to do something to show her support. Her soccer team, the Blue Blitz, wanted to help our family.

She said the soccer team had changed their name to Blue Blitz for Brittany. They had prepared a special container to collect money for our family. Every time their team made a goal, they passed the container around to the people on the sidelines.

For a moment, I was speechless. You hear human interest stories on the news about how people reach out, but it's different when you are the one being helped. She said they still had a number of games to play, and she would bring the container when they had finished the season.

My voice cracked as I said, "Thank you so much, Nancy. Please thank your daughter and her teammates for the kindness they are showing my family. Let them know how much we appreciate them extending their love to us."

"I sure will," she said.

"Thank you again," I replied. "We'll keep in touch."

When you are so moved by something, it's impossible to convey your thanks strongly enough. While we were there in the hospital, these girls were out on the field trying their best to make a goal so they could pass around the bucket on behalf of our Brittany. Every time they played, she was in their thoughts. How do you properly thank someone for a gift like that?

A couple days later, a nurse came in with a newspaper and asked if we had read the article about the girls' soccer team in Irvine. We knew who she was talking about, but didn't expect an article to be in the paper.

The nurse said, "Here, I marked it for you. You have so many people looking out for you." She smiled as she walked away.

The article read:

> *"A girls' all-star soccer team in South Irvine is donating money to help pay the hospital bills for a 4-year-old girl from Costa Mesa who has been diagnosed with leukemia. The Blue Blitz, which consists of fifteen 8 and 9 year old girls, was inspired to help Brittany Engle when they read an article about her in the newspaper. One of the girls, Kaley Pickett, was worried when her parents showed her the article to let her know how fortunate she was to be healthy and able to play soccer. Kaley and the other girls decided to dedicate their season to Brittany. Also, the parents decided that each player would contribute $1 for every goal the team scored and an additional $1 for every shout-out. The girls earned money from their parents by doing chores and helping with household tasks. The coach was very proud of his team for wanting to contribute to such a worthy cause and said they were glad to be able to do something for someone who is not able to play soccer or lead a normal life."*

What a tribute to a remarkable girl. This was not the last we would be hearing from Kaley and her mother, Nancy.

ANOTHER ROSE

That evening while resting in bed, my phone rang. I checked the display before picking it up. It was my sister in New York. I had been updating her almost daily on what was going on. I depended on her, more than she knew, to keep me from falling apart. Some family members can be therapy for your soul.

I picked up the phone and said, "Hi, Dorothy."

"Hi, how is everything going?" she asked.

"Well, we haven't seen too much change the last few days," I answered.

"Don't get discouraged," she said. "I know someone who might be able to help."

In a surprised voice I asked, "Who? What do you mean?"

She went on to tell me that a friend of hers in New York was a psychic who did readings over the phone and who could send healing power from a distance. She told me they had had a long conversation about Brittany and that she would love to send her healing powers our way if we wanted her to. I was moved by the fact that someone so far away who didn't know us would take the time to do this.

"What's her name?" I asked.

There was a short pause before she answered. "I think this will surprise you. Her name is Rose."

"Rose?" I asked. "Her name is Rose?" I couldn't believe my ears.

"Yes," my sister answered.

"Oh, yes, you tell her yes. We would love to have her help us."

"You know, Dorothy," I continued. "I've been going through some things that are making me think about stuff I've never thought about before."

"What do you mean?" she asked. I went on to tell her about the sunbeams, the medallion Lori found, the pink roses in the garden, the three women who came into our lives, and everything that was happening as a result of the *L.A. Times* article. I ended by saying, "I don't know what to make of it all."

She reminded me, "You've always been one to pay attention to detail and believe things happen for a reason. You're the one who always says there are no coincidences, and I believe that, too."

"Yes, thank you for reminding me. I'm doing my best to hang in there and stay positive."

Her next words were, "Never stop believing."

I always felt better when I talked to her. She understood me and always encouraged the positive.

"Thanks, Dorothy, for bringing Rose into our life. Please tell her how grateful we are for her kindness."

I wasn't sure what to expect, but every day I found myself hoping that Rose's healing energy would come forth from New York and work a miracle. Sometimes when Brittany was sleeping, I would sit and wonder what Rose was doing at that moment. I would close my eyes and try to feel her spirit working. I would sit on one side of Brittany's bed and imagine Rose sitting across from me. I could see us working together to bring healing power down from heaven. In my mind, I could see her face, and she always had a slight smile and a warm glow in her eyes. I couldn't tell if it was working for Brittany, but I knew it was giving me comfort.

Many people believe we are all God's children and are all one. Although our lives are different and we live all over the planet, we all have the same basic needs and share the same feelings. Our experiences are different, but we share the same essence of life. We all want to love and be loved. If we are all one, then any one of us could send our energy to anyone, anywhere, at anytime.

If you were out in space looking back at Earth, you would see the world differently. It would be easy to imagine a mist of loveliness wrapped around our planet, making everyone content with life.

A SETBACK

I came to the hospital one morning with my hopes high, but as I walked into the room, I saw four doctors standing around Brittany's bed. My heart sank. Lori was standing in the corner, still and silent. My heart was racing as I hurried over to her. As I passed the doctors, I caught a glimpse of Brittany's face. Her eyes were closed, but she appeared to be breathing. I could see the doctors were picking at something around her stomach.

I hugged my daughter and asked in a fearful tone, "What's going on?"

She said, "Well, the fungus has caused the tissue around her intestine to die, which caused the surrounding area to bleed. It formed a giant blood clot on her stomach. For the last half hour, they have been slowly removing it, bit by bit. They said they have to go slowly so they don't cause more bleeding."

"Oh, Lori. Does this mean the new medicine isn't working? Did they expect this to happen?"

Her voice was cracking as she said, "I don't know, Mom. No one has said anything yet."

I walked over as close as I could and peeked between the doctors' shoulders. After watching for a few minutes, I could tell it was going to be a long process. They must have knocked Brittany out because she didn't move at all and her eyes stayed closed.

About an hour later, they had finished and put a bandage over the area. Not knowing what to expect was always the hardest part. Would it happen again? Would the skin grow back? Would her body work the way it was supposed to? Despite the fear we felt, we never stopped hoping for a miracle.

It's human nature to always search for a reason to be optimistic. This is a gift from our Creator. Our hearts will always hang on dearly to the smallest possibility of seeing a miracle. Our souls won't let us release this thought. It becomes a part of us.

As the doctors were leaving, one came over and said, "This was something we didn't expect, but we have removed the clot and bandaged her up. Now, we have to wait and see. As you know, we are treating her separately for two types of diseases. It's tough, but we are still hopeful."

Lori responded in a broken voice, "But, how will we know it's really working? When will we know if she's getting better?" It was heartbreaking to hear her say these words.

The doctor hesitated for a moment before answering. To me, that hesitation meant he was trying to figure how to say what he had to say in a positive way.

He lifted his head and said, "We just don't know. This is a new drug and her situation is complicated. We are doing all we can. Unfortunately, we just have to wait and see." He patted her on the shoulder then turned and walked away.

I hugged Lori tightly and let her cry. I tried not to make a sound as the tears rolled down my face. I didn't have a good feeling about things. It was a struggle to stay positive, but I knew I had to. After a few minutes, we sat down and tried to relax.

"Where is Gary?" I asked.

"His van broke down, Mom," Lori answered. "He thinks it's the clutch. He went to get some parts and is going to fix it himself in the parking lot."

"Oh, dear," I said. I took a deep breath and lowered my head. The weight of all this was so heavy. Sometimes it felt like it was pushing us down into the ground. "How about I go see how he's doing. If he's hungry, I'll go get him something. Do you want anything?"

"No, I'm fine," she answered. "Go ahead, I'll get something later."

I sat down and took her hands and gave them a squeeze. I knew she wanted to just lie down and cry. It's so frustrating when there's nothing you can say or do to bring back that spark of hope when you are continually getting bad news.

"Do you want to go with me?" I asked.

"No. I want to stay here with Brittany."

"OK. I'll be back in just a little bit. Try to stretch out and get some rest."

I went outside to look for Gary. It took a while, but I finally found him in the parking lot at the Ronald McDonald House across the street. There, beside his car, was the engine. He had taken the engine out right there in the parking lot and was working to repair whatever was wrong.

"Wow, I hope you know what you're doing," I said with a laugh.

We both laughed as he said, "Yeah, I do. Don't worry." I watched for a minute and then asked if he was hungry.

"I'm starving," he answered.

"Well, what sounds good?" I asked.

"Any kind of sandwich and a big cold drink would be great," he answered. He seemed to be in control of his emotions, but I knew inside he was struggling to hang on.

When I returned with the food, a security guard was watching him. Someone had complained about him making a mess in the parking lot.

"How long do you think it will take you?" the guard asked.

"I'm working as fast as I can. I'm sorry for dirtying up the place, but I promise to clean it all up when I'm done. It might be another hour."

The guard smiled at us both and said, "Well, good luck. Just don't leave a mess." Then he turned and walked away. Gary kept on working as I filled him in on what was happening at the hospital. Every now and then, he would stop and listen more intently. His medical background was probably helping him fill in the gaps. He stayed calm, but I knew he was hurting.

"I'm going to head back to the hospital. Is there anything else you need?" I asked.

In his normal, calm voice he said, "I'm good for now. I'll be about another half hour or so; then I'll come over."

I gave him a hug and said, "Hang in there." Patting him on the back, I said with a smile, "Don't forget to eat."

As I walked away, I suddenly realized he hadn't had a moment yet to share anything about all he had been through in Saudi Arabia. His job in the war put him right in middle of fear and pain. I could only imagine how haunting some of those memories could be. As I stopped and looked back, I wondered if he was holding in a tremendous amount of pain so it wouldn't distract him from being there for his daughter. His best friends were still in the Middle East and he had no clue of their status. I worried that he might be holding in dark moments without anyone even knowing how he felt.

Back at the room, I filled Lori in on how the car situation was coming along. I also asked if she had shown Brittany the medallion and the picture of Sai Baba.

"Yes, I did, last night," she answered. "She wanted to hold the medallion, and she wanted me to take the picture off the wall and give it to her. When I gave her the picture, she held it to her chest. I asked her if she knew who it was, and she told me yes."

"You're kidding," I said in a shocked voice. "How would she know this man?"

"I don't know, Mom, but she said she did. She seemed content so I didn't ask questions. After she held the medallion for a while, she motioned for me to hang it back up, and then she just lay there with her eyes closed, holding the picture to her chest."

"Maybe she thought it was someone else," I said. "The morphine could be making her confused."

"I don't know, Mom. Sometimes she feels so sure of herself. It scares me a little," she said.

"Why does that scare you?" I asked.

"Well," she answered, "it makes me wonder if she is connecting with souls on the other side and maybe talking with angels. The thought of her talking with those on the other side makes me think she is going there and I'm not ready for her to go, Mom. I don't want to lose her." I wasn't sure what to say. We both stood there with tears in our eyes.

We sat down and began talking about what we did and didn't believe in, and what we thought might be possible. Who can say for sure what the universe is about and what we, as human beings, are capable of? There is so much written about the power of the mind and the ties we have with the spiritual world. There are so many beliefs about where we came from, why we are here, and what happens when we die. We each have to decide for ourselves what we believe in, what makes sense, and what gives us comfort.

As Lori and I stretched out in our chairs and tried to take a nap, my mind drifted back to when I was a teenager, to the night before I left home for the first time to go to college. As I lay there with my eyes closed, I remembered the conversation I had with my dad that night.

I sat on the edge of my bed staring at the floor with my hands folded in my lap. I could hear my father coming down the hall. As his footsteps came closer, I waited to see if he was going to stop or walk by. Not to my surprise, he stopped and peeked in. He asked if he could sit down and I nodded yes. I knew he was going to pat me on the knee. He always did that.

His arm moved around my shoulders and pulled me close. My head automatically leaned toward that comfort spot below his chin and complete serenity wrapped around me. We talked for almost an hour about life's ups and downs, about making friends, being kind, using good judgment and most of all, believing in yourself. Finally when we were both talked out, he patted my knee, stood up, looked down at me and said:

"Your beliefs will carry you through. It doesn't matter what you believe in, just believe in something. If it gives you peace of mind, then it's right for you. Be strong and don't let anyone bamboozle you."

At the time, it seemed like a lot to think about, so after he left, I quickly wrote it down. It was just a few sentences, but I knew if I took time to ponder it, I would understand the impact of his words. Down deep inside, where I can't even reach, these words were kept safe for me. Now, they would come back to me and help me in this trying time. Thank you, Daddy.

It took Gary half the day to complete the repair on his car, but when he was done, the van started right up. He went to the Ronald McDonald House to get cleaned up before coming back to the hospital.

When he returned, I asked, "Is the van working OK?"

"Yep," he answered. "It's working great now." He smiled and went over to see his little girl, and she perked up when she saw him. They sat together and talked about the letters and pictures they had sent back and forth while he was away. She loved hearing his stories. They talked for almost an hour before she dozed off.

Code Blue

While Brittany slept, we each got comfortable and closed our eyes, hoping to get a short nap. Within minutes, we were jolted out of our half-asleep state by a loud beeping. We sat up immediately and watched as a nurse went running down the hall yelling "Code Blue . . . Code Blue!" I had never heard that in real life before, but remembered seeing it on TV. In hospital dramas, it meant someone had stopped breathing. Several nurses came running down the hall. One was pushing a big machine and it looked like they were coming to our room.

We looked at Brittany to see if something was wrong, but she lay quietly with her eyes closed and didn't appear to be in any kind of distress. Was the monitor telling the nurses' station something was wrong that we couldn't see? Panic struck like a knife. As the nurse pushing the machine came closer, she ran past our room to the room next to us. We were instantly relived, but our hearts ached for the child in the next room.

The hospital staff was moving so fast. My heart was pounding because I knew this meant a child might die. It's different in person than it is on TV. Anxiety seeps into every vein and terror stops you dead.

Three people ran out of the room and stood against the wall in the hallway. They looked like the mother, grandmother, and brother. They were all crying as they huddled together with their arms around each other. We stood like statues watching them through the window. They were terrified. None of us moved an inch. We just stared at those people and watched their faces. It was so frightening. After about ten minutes, a nurse came out and motioned for the family to go back in.

My daughter sat down in a chair and put her face in her hands and began to cry. I went over and put my arms around her shoulders. I knew what she was thinking.

"Oh, Mom," she cried. "What if this happens to Brittany? What if she stops breathing?"

"It's not going to happen to Brittany. Look at her. She's resting comfortably."

As brave a soul as Gary was, I could see he was frightened as he stood over Brittany's bed. He stroked her arm as a few tears rolled slowly down his cheek.

I walked out into the hall and stood against the far wall and looked into the neighboring room. I saw the little boy's eyes were open. His mother smiled as she stroked his forehead. I couldn't help but wonder what was going through this child's mind right then. Did he go to heaven for a few moments? I had read that when someone dies and then is revived, many times the person gets a glimpse of heaven.

It's difficult to express what happens when you see all this up close. You can't truly comprehend the fear and anxiety unless you experience it yourself. I couldn't bring myself to imagine this happening to Brittany. I tried to push it out of my mind, but I knew it was possible. I leaned against the wall and closed my eyes and said, "No, God. No! Please. This is not going to happen to us. Brittany is going to be fine because I am going to pray like I've never prayed before."

When I opened my eyes, I saw my daughter staring through the window, waiting for a sign. I smiled and gave a thumbs-up to let her and Gary know the boy was OK. The seriousness of our situation had just become much more real.

That night I thanked God for forcing me to see how important it is to treasure every moment of life.

CHURCH WITH DAWN

Dawn had asked several times if I wanted to meet her for church one Sunday morning. I didn't really want to, but I felt I should, after all she had been doing for us. So, that Sunday I got up, got ready, and went. She had told me where she and her husband always sat, and when I got there, it only took a moment to spot them. I walked over to the end of their aisle and gave a short wave to get her attention. She waved back and pointed to an empty spot on the pew beside her. Once I was seated and comfortable, she introduced me to her husband, who seemed to know who I was. I have to admit, it felt good to be there.

Beautiful music played as a few stragglers made their way in. As the music played, children came walking in from the back, on both sides of the chapel, up to the front. There were about fifteen on each side, aged five to eight. Dawn leaned over and explained that every Sunday they marched in, lined up at the front of the church, and sang at the beginning of the service. There's nothing as heartwarming as the sound of sweet little voices singing. As I listened, I imagined our little Brittany standing there singing with them. I couldn't help but get teary-eyed. Their sound was captivating and soothing. My heart felt full. It was both sweet and sad at the same time. When they were done, they marched back out and went to their Sunday school class.

All I could think of was Brittany and how wonderful it would be to see her standing there singing. Dawn saw it was difficult for me so she reached over and touched my arm and smiled. She was such a sweet person. When the service was over, I thanked her for inviting me. As we hugged, she said she would see me soon. Part of me couldn't wait to go back the following Sunday, and part of me never wanted to go again. Driving away I broke down and asked God again why this was happening to Brittany. Why do little children have to suffer?

When I got to the hospital, I sat in my car thinking about all the children inside and all the parents and other family members who were asking God the same question. This is only one hospital out of thousands all over the world where the same events go on continually. We all know that people are born and people die every day. It's the circle of life, but why do some suffer more than others? I don't know if we will ever get the answer to that question. There has to be some way to look at life and death without it seeming so tragic.

Our Little Valentine

When February 14 arrived, it was hard to believe that it was already Valentine's Day. Everyone loves Valentine's Day because it's a day for showing people how much they mean to us. I remembered my kids being little and buying those little packages of Valentine's Day cards for all their classmates. We would sit at the dining room table the night before the school Valentine's Day party, with all the cards spread out and divided, one group for boys and one group for girls, and then they would pick the ones they liked the most for their best friends. At school, they had already made a special Valentine's box that would hold all the cards and candies from their classmates. The parents made cookies and other goodies for the kids to take to school. That's what Brittany would have been doing with her friends at her new school, but instead, we had our own little party at the hospital.

Kat brought Brittany a beautiful unicorn music box. It was round and about eight inches high. It would turn like a carousel as the music played. I immediately noticed the little square mirrors all around the bottom. Brittany hadn't seen herself in a mirror since her hair started falling out, and I was afraid she would catch a glimpse of herself and start crying.

As Lori handed it to her, her eyes brightened. She turned the key and the song *Somewhere over the Rainbow* began to play. She had always loved that song. Her little lips smiled and she stared intently as the carousel went round and round. It was a magical moment.

I wanted to cry as I watched her holding the beautiful box and listening to the music. Although she looked content and somewhat happy, I thought my heart was going to burst. Even though I was caught up in the magic, I still couldn't stop worrying that she would see herself in the mirrors and notice that she had lost almost all her hair, but she never said a thing. She never complained or cried. She just quietly lay there enjoying the music. What a perfect gift.

How Could This Happen

When I arrived that morning, Brittany was sleeping and Lori was sitting in the corner reading. I noticed Gary wasn't in the room and asked Lori where he was.

"A nurse came and got him a while ago," she said. "He had a phone call from his family."

"Well," I said, "they probably called to see how Brittany was doing. I'm sure it's hard for him to talk about it."

About an hour and a half had passed since he had left. It wasn't like him to leave for this long without letting Lori know when he would be back, so she decided to go looking for him. She went to the nurses' station and asked one of the nurses, "Do you happen to know where Gary went? He came here to get a phone call and has been gone for a while."

The nurse pointed down the hall and said, "When he hung up, he seemed upset. He walked away without saying anything. There's a porch at the end of the hall, maybe he's there."

Lori walked to the end of the hall and out to the porch. There he was, sitting in the far corner with his face in his hands. She walked over and sat down beside him.

"What's wrong, Gary?" she asked.

In a broken voice he answered, "My sister Arlynne was killed in a car accident."

"Oh, Gary, what happened?" she said.

"She and Mike had just gotten engaged. They were on their way back from Phoenix and had a blowout on the rear tire and the truck flipped. Her head hit the roof as the car landed, and she was killed."

This was absolutely crushing news. Gary was from a family of seven children, and Arlynne was his favorite sister. He sat in shock while Lori did her best to console him. You want to scream at God and ask, "Why?" but you know there is no answer to that question. I felt terrible, but didn't know what to do. There just isn't any way to take away the pain.

The next few days were extremely tough for Gary. He wanted to go to Utah for his sister's funeral and be with his family during that devastating time, but he was afraid to leave Brittany. It was heart-rending to watch him battling with the question of whether to stay or go. He was so afraid that if he left, Brittany wouldn't be there when he came back. Finally, he made a decision and told Lori he felt it best to stay with Brittany.

Lori and I didn't know what to do to help Gary. How do you ease the pain of such a tragedy? How do you make it not hurt so much? All the comforting words you can think of are not enough, but we did our best. All of us still had a battle to fight, and all good soldiers must rise up, and he did his best

KIND HEARTS REACH OUT

That morning, we got a call from Nancy Pickett, the mother of Kaley, the girl on the soccer team. She asked if she and two of her friends could come and pray for Brittany. People often told us they were sending prayers our way, but these women wanted to be in

Brittany's presence and make it more personal. We were quite moved by this and welcomed them.

The next afternoon, they arrived around two o'clock. Nancy introduced us to her friends, and we thanked them for taking time out of their day to do this.

"How are the girls doing with their games?" I asked Nancy.

She explained, "They made it to the finals, which are on March 3rd, so we'll see."

"Wow, that's wonderful." I replied. "They must be so excited."

Then she added, "Having a good cause to fight for has made this season one to remember."

"Well," I said, "knowing they are fighting for us is something we will never forget."

Before they prayed, Nancy asked, "Do you mind if we use our rosaries?"

"Of course not," Lori answered with a smile. "Thank you for caring so much."

They held hands in a circle over Brittany and began their prayers. We stood in reverence and watched as they prayed for her healing and asked that our family be comforted. It was a beautiful prayer filled with honest love.

Three wonderful, caring souls wrapped their arms around us that day. It was plain to see that the phrase "by giving, you receive" was well taught in Kaley's home. Moments like these strengthened my belief that we all share in a universal force that connects us all through the spirit of love.

As they were leaving, we hugged each of them and thanked them for taking the time to come and be there for us.

TALKING WITH ANGELS

So much had happened so quickly over the last month and a half. It was hard to believe that so much time had passed. All Brittany's activities—coloring, watching TV, having conversations with Rose the bear, and other communication—were minimal now. Most of the time, she was sedated and asleep. Her body was wearing out.

When I came that day, I asked Lori if anything had changed. She gave me a solemn look and told me that she had asked Brittany if she had seen angels. I was afraid to hear the answer, but I asked, "What did she say?"

Lori replied, "She said yes."

That was frightening to hear. "What do you think that means?" I asked.

"I'm not sure. Many times this week, after she had been sleeping for a while, Brittany woke up and told me she had been talking with angels. I don't know if that means they are coming for her or if they are telling her to keep fighting."

I put my arms around her as we both shed a few tears. We weren't sure what it meant, but we were beginning to realize that Brittany might not make it. Letting in the thought was still almost impossible. You tell yourself you need to accept it so you can prepare to deal with it, but it's so hard to let that wall down.

Later that evening, Kat came when no one was there, so we didn't know what took place until we saw her the next day. This is what she told us:

Brittany told me about a woman that would come and visit her. She would sit at the foot of her bed or stand by her head. She said she knew her, and felt comfortable with her, but didn't know her name. When I asked her what she looked like, the only thing she said was that she had red hair.

Kat asked Lori, "Do you know anyone with red hair? Do you have any idea who this woman is that comes to visit her?"

Lori was stunned. In a choked voice she answered, "Gary's sister, Arlynne, the one who recently passed away, had red hair." It was such a jolt that it was almost impossible to even react.

If it was Arlynne, was she there to help Brittany to the other side or to tell her not to give up? Our minds were torn between what we wanted to believe and what we knew may be the truth.

Kat also told us that a few days before, Brittany had said Jesus was talking to her. When she asked her what He said, Brittany had closed her eyes and gone to sleep. Kat said that then the most amazing feeling came over her. She sensed that Brittany was sitting in a beautiful bright light, filled with love and energy. What did all this mean?

THE BLUE BLITZ PLAYOFFS

As the end of their season approached, the Blue Blitz for Brittany soccer team had contributed almost $500. Kaley and her mom came to our house and presented me with the money. That moment was so heartwarming. We're used to everyone being so caught up in the things they have to do in their own lives. To see people taking time to extend themselves to complete strangers was quite something.

"Thank you so much for your kindness," I said. "I don't know how we can ever thank you enough. Our entire family has been deeply touched, and from what I read in the paper, your kindness has touched many others as well." We shared hugs and some tears before they went on their way.

Many times during the last month, I had thought of them out on the field making goals, cheering, and passing around the bucket. Each person at the game knew they were making their own personal contribution to our cause. I imagined being one of the people sitting in the stands and how good my heart would feel when I dropped my money in. This goodwill spread to many people and gave them all a chance to receive the wonderful feeling of sharing what's in ones heart.

On March 3rd, I went to the playoffs and watched the girls play their hardest. It was exhilarating to hear people cheering for them. When the game was over, I asked if the team could come and sit with me for a minute. We gathered on a grassy spot away from the crowd. I couldn't help getting teary-eyed as I thanked them all for caring about our family. I wanted them to remember this for the rest of their lives, so I had made them a special gift.

"I made something for each of you," I said. "I hope it will always remind you of what you did to make a difference in someone else's life. We will never forget you."

As I handed out the gifts, I saw some tears. The gift was a small double-sided picture frame. On one side was a picture of Brittany and on the other side was a poem. As they sat on the grass looking at Brittany's picture, I read the poem.

Love shows in so many ways. Those who love will always see it.

It speaks in so many voices. Those who love will always hear it.

Love is for so many reasons. Those who love will never ask why.

It was difficult to read without crying, because I could see how it touched them.

"How is Brittany doing?" one of the girls asked.

I didn't want to explain the details, so I just said, "It's tough right now, but she's a fighter."

We shared some hugs and they wished us the best. For those few moments, I felt we were all wrapped in the wings of angels.

Blue Blitz for Brittany didn't win the championship that year, but they accomplished something far greater, something they would remember for the rest of their life.

Chapter Three

A Test of Strength

DISNEYLAND

On March 10th, Brittany would turn five years old. We had planned to take her to Disneyland, but as her birthday got closer, we could see this would be impossible. Instead, my daughter and I decided to go and take pictures, and then show them to Brittany on her birthday. It wouldn't be exactly like being there, but it was the best we could do. Gary stayed with Brittany while we were gone. It was good for them to have some time alone.

At Disneyland we took videos of everything. Every time we saw a Disney character, we asked for their picture. We told them about Brittany and asked if they would wave and say something to her. Of course, they were more than happy to.

Like all little girls, Brittany loved dressing up. Her favorite movie was *The Little Mermaid,* so we wanted to find something from that movie to take back to her. We went to the Disney Store on Main Street and looked at many things, wondering which one would cheer her up and make her feel that she was a part of the world. Then we saw it, a Little Mermaid dress! It was perfect! We knew she would love it.

We were excited to get back to the hospital and show her the dress. As we were driving back, I wondered if she would be able to open her eyes and see it. Then, I realized how sad she might feel if she couldn't put it on. Were we doing the right thing, to get her excited only to hang the dress someplace where she could only look at it, and not feel it on her body and see how pretty she looked?

Again, I had to tighten my jaw to keep the tears from flowing. Is there going to be a moment when we have to accept the worse? You try to be strong because that's what people expect you to do. That's what your family needs you to do. Your arms are supposed to be the ones that comfort and console. Your words are supposed to be the ones that bring hope. Inside you want to crumble in despair, but you can't.

We parked the car and started walking toward the hospital. The closer we got, the faster we walked. I was excited, but still my heart ached at the thought that the dress might make her sad.

When we walked into the room, the nurses were at her bedside doing something. Whenever we saw more than one nurse our hearts would stop. When they heard us come in, they turned toward us. Tons of weight lifted when we saw their smiles. Every time you leave and come back you go through the same things. You worry constantly that something bad might happen when you're not there.

So much had happened to Brittany's little body in the last month and a half. She rarely opened her eyes anymore. As Lori stood there with the dress, Gary tapped on Brittany's arm. I leaned down close to her ear and said, "We have something for you that you will love." As her eyes opened, Lori held the dress up so she could see the whole thing. Her eyes popped open wide and a beautiful smile lit up her face as Lori pointed out the picture of Ariel, the Little Mermaid, on the front. I will never forget the excitement in her eyes. We couldn't believe how alert she became.

For the first time in days, she spoke. She asked if she could put it on. I looked at Lori and Gary, and then at the nurse. I wasn't sure what to say. The nurse smiled and nodded, yes. With all the tubes coming out of her body it wasn't easy, but with the nurses' help, Lori and Gary got her into the dress. I could see that their hearts were breaking. I was torn apart. Part of me was filled with happiness, while another part cried because I knew how much Brittany would love to jump up and dance around the room in her beautiful dress.

For now, we were just happy she was able to lie there feeling like a little Princess. Her hand moved slowly over the bodice as she tried to tilt her head enough to see how it flared out across her tiny legs. She smiled and said in her soft little voice, "It's so pretty." It was amazing how this lifted her spirits, even if it was only for a few moments.

She didn't want to take it off, so we left it on. As she drifted off to sleep, I closed my eyes and prayed, "Please God, let her dream of dancing in her pretty dress."

ANOTHER TEST OF FAITH

When I got to the hospital room the next day, Lori quickly came over to me, took my arm, and pulled me into the hallway. Immediately I felt sick inside because she had never done this before. I could see sadness in her face and knew it meant something had happened.

"Mom," she said. "Gary got more bad news today."

"Oh, Lori, what's happened this time?" I asked.

"His cousin and uncle were killed in a car accident yesterday. His mom called him this morning. He's over at the Ronald McDonald House right now."

"Oh, Lori, how can so much happen at the same time? This is terrible. How is he?"

"Not too good right now," she answered. "He's so upset. His family is having such a difficult time. It hasn't been that long since his sister was killed, so this is a lot for them. He thinks he should be there with his family."

"I can understand that. What do you think he'll do?" I asked.

"Brittany isn't improving, so I think he'll stay. He would feel terrible if he left and she wasn't here when he came back."

My heart went out to him. This was such a heavy load to bear, and I knew it was tearing him apart. He wanted to be with his family, but was afraid to leave his little girl. How could we possibly help ease his pain? It was just too much.

Later that evening, he came back to the hospital and told us he had decided to stay with Brittany. We knew what a hard decision that must have been. We couldn't get the big question "WHY?" out of our heads. The emotions connected to all of this were almost too much to bear. There was so much heartache.

I stood numbly in the corner and prayed, "Please God, wrap your arms around Gary and let him know his loved ones are in a good place."

The next morning, right after I arrived, three attendants came in pushing a gurney. I panicked at the thought of what that meant. Lori grabbed my arm and pulled me to the side.

"Lori, what's happening?" I asked. I could hardly breathe.

"Her kidneys are failing. They are going to have to put tubes in both kidneys so they can drain."

"Oh, no," I said, as I began to cry. "What does this mean, Lori?"

Her voice was broken as she said, "Things aren't looking good, Mom." I hugged her close and we both cried quietly. Brittany was almost lifeless as they moved her to the gurney. As they passed us, we saw her eyes were closed. Was she aware of what was going on? Was she afraid? Was she at peace, talking with angels?

A few hours later, they brought her back. She was sleeping and would sleep for a good while more. Lori and Gary said they had an appointment with the doctor and they would be back in a while, so I pulled up a chair close to Brittany's bed and laid my head next to hers on the pillow.

My mind drifted back to a time when Brittany and I were in my car. This had been about a year ago when she just turned four. I don't remember where we were going, but I remember I was really angry at something that was going on in my life. It's funny, but sometimes I talked to her as if she were an adult. She seemed to have such good answers to my questions, and I was always curious to hear what she might say. I told her what I was angry about and asked her what she would do. Her answer was, "You just have to deal with it." Well, there you go, I thought. I looked at her and laughed. She looked back at me and said, "Don't worry about it, it will be OK." I remember saying, "But, it's not OK. It makes me mad." With raised eyebrows, she looked at me again and said only, "Grandma!" I laughed and said, "OK."

Brittany had just been so cute about it all. I smiled to myself thinking how glad I was to be able to be with her while she was growing up. I thought . . . here is this amazing little person sitting next to me, giving me advice. I reached over and patted her on the knee and said, "I love you so much." She turned her head, smiled back, and said, "I love you more."

She learned that little phrase from her mother. They would always say that to each other. I think it is the sweetest thing ever.

HAPPY BIRTHDAY BRITTANY

Though our plans had been to take her to Disneyland for her birthday party, instead, Disneyland came to Brittany. After making sure she was awake, the nurses surprised us with pink balloons and a cake with five pink candles. Brittany smiled a tiny smile as we sang Happy Birthday to her. Lori and Gary held the cake close to her as they blew out the candles. Then, Lori took one of the balloons and moved close to her hands. She reached up just enough to barely tap the balloon into the air. I can't believe how excited we got just to see her tap that balloon. It was only a brief moment, but it made me think she was still fighting.

We started the Disneyland video, but in just a few minutes, she was starting to nod off. We watched the video for a short while and then turned it off. It was for Brittany, and she couldn't watch it. We felt so bad, we just couldn't continue watching.

After the party, Lori and Gary left to speak with the doctors. When they came back, they walked over to Brittany's bed and just stood there watching her sleep. I was going to ask what the doctors said, but a nurse came in to take vital signs so we all stepped away. At the same time, Kat came in and started talking to Lori and Gary, so I sat down in a chair and let them talk. I didn't see fear in anyone's face. There was a different air in the room which gave me an odd feeling about what was going on, a feeling that scared me.

HOLD ME TIGHT

Most of the time now, Brittany was heavily sedated and didn't move or open her eyes much. I knew that couldn't be a good thing, but hoped her body was healing during this time. I've been told that when our body is at rest, this is when it does its repairing.

As I stood over her, I was surprised to see her lips moving. It looked like she was trying to speak. I couldn't understand what she was saying and this upset me terribly. Was she trying to say something to me, or was she speaking with Jesus or angels again? I wanted to know what she was saying. Was she saying, "I'm scared" or "Don't worry, I'll be all right, Grandma"? Was she afraid, or was she at peace? I leaned over and told her I didn't understand what she said and asked her to say it again, but she didn't respond. That broke my heart and for a second I panicked. I wanted to know if she was afraid, but she laid quiet again and now I would never know. That was so hard to deal with.

Lori got comfortable in the corner chair next to Gary so that she could rest while Kat did some healing work. Kat walked over to the bed and, as she often did, raised her hands over Brittany. As she closed her eyes to begin the healing work, suddenly Brittany woke up, sat straight up in bed, and said, "No, no." Then she fell back into an unconscious state.

Extremely startled, we all stood up and looked at Kat, waiting for her to respond. What we had just witnessed had never happened before. Brittany had always been open to receiving what Kat was doing.

In a panic, Lori asked Kat, "What just happened?"

Though to us it was completely unexpected, it didn't surprise Kat quite as much because she felt all along that Brittany was in charge at a deep level. Kat told Lori, "Healing is not just about the body. Healing is also preparation for the soul, for what comes in the next life. I think Brittany was trying to tell us where she is headed."

"What do you mean?" Lori asked.

There was a short pause as Kat chose her next words carefully. "Well," she answered, "Brittany wants us to stop trying to heal her."

We all just stood there, unable to react. We didn't know what to say or do. How do you decide to stop trying to heal someone you love? How do you know it's the right decision? We were stunned into silence as we thought about what we needed to do next.

Kat, Barbara, and Dawn had always sensed that in reality, Brittany was guiding them along. Early on, Barbara had said that she felt Brittany had called them into a sacred contract. She explained that a sacred contract is a contract with God, saying this is the family I'm going to work with, and this is the work I am going to do. Kat had said that what she was learning from Brittany was preparing her for work with others to come. All three felt their experience with Brittany had much to do with her own transition to the afterlife.

Trying to envision Brittany well was impossible now. All the sickness and side effects from the treatments had taken their toll and it was all too much for her. Her body was shutting down, and Brittany knew it better than any of us.

That night, a nurse came in with equipment to give Brittany her usual breathing treatment. When she approached her bed, Lori stopped her. I jumped up and said in a startled voice, "But she needs it, Lori."

Lori, Gary, and Kat all looked at me without speaking. Their eyes told the tale. This was it. I sank into the chair and put my face in my hands and cried as I realized tonight we were losing her. I don't even know how to explain the heartache we all felt.

Lori came over and put her arm around me and said, "Mom, nothing in her body is working anymore. She would be on life support with no hope of every regaining consciousness. It's too much for her. Remember when she said she was talking with angels and she saw Gary's sister? She knew, Mom. She knew she was going. None of us want to lose her, but she's going."

"Oh, Lori," I said with tears flowing down my face. "I can't believe this is happening." I could barely get the words out.

I knew how much it hurt Lori and Gary to see Brittany like this. Their hearts were breaking, and I knew I couldn't take away their pain.

Without a word to each other, we all got up and stood in a circle around the bed while Brittany lay there in a coma. We stretched our hands out across her and then all of a sudden, Brittany sat straight up, pushed our hands away, and lay back down, unconscious again. We were in shock and just stared at each other in silence. At that moment, we had no doubt that Brittany knew much more than we did and was ready to move on to the next part of her journey.

The next few minutes were agonizing as we sat staring at the equipment monitoring Brittany's vital signs. The most heart-rending moment came when a nurse asked Lori if she wanted to hold Brittany. I could see the fear in Lori's eyes as she thought for a moment. Finally, she said yes. Oh my God, I thought. This will crush her. I couldn't even imagine how she felt at that moment.

Two nurses began removing tubes from Brittany's body. It was horrible to watch. I could hardly breathe as I watched all the life saving equipment being taken from her, leaving only what monitored her heart.

Lori sat in the chair and waited for the nurse to place Brittany her in her arms as Gary stood next to her. There was no way to hold back the tears and no way to describe the pain we felt. As Lori held her, I noticed a steadying of her heartbeat on the monitor. I knew that meant Brittany was feeling her mother's arms holding her . . . for her last few moments, she felt her mother's love, and it calmed her. Gary reached over and grasped Brittany's little hand in his. They were quietly saying their goodbyes.

After about fifteen minutes, Lori asked that they put her back in her bed. She felt they had said what they needed to say to each other. She was afraid of what it would feel like to hold Brittany when all her life was gone.

My father had passed away just a year earlier and as I stood beside her bed with tears running down my face, I closed my eyes and said, "Daddy, bring our Brittany home and take good care of her." A few minutes passed then we saw the lines on the monitor go flat. We were engulfed in silence.

If you have been through this, you know how enormous the emotional anguish of that moment is. Nothing you have ever experienced feels so final. Lori, bless her heart, climbed into the bed and lay next to Brittany as Gary stood beside the bed holding her hand. No one was able to hold back their tears. I remember thinking even then that if I prayed hard enough, God would bring her back. As I prayed with all my heart, I watched to see if her chest would start to move up and down as she began to breathe again, but she didn't. She was really gone.

Before leaving that night, we dressed Brittany in her new pajamas, the ones that were covered in little pink roses, and the slippers with pink roses that her Grandma Melba had made for her. Finally, she looked at peace.

It was hard for us to leave the hospital without her. Walking away seemed wrong, but there was nothing left for us to do. The nurse said they would take care of everything.

Kat told us that in the traditional Chinese belief system, when someone dies, the Yin and Yang separate. The Yin goes back to Mother Earth, and the Yang goes on to heaven. There is a tearing apart. This was our first experience in feeling the tearing apart.

BRITTANY'S SERVICE

The service for Brittany was held at the Golden Circle Church, the church Dawn had taken me to. Friends and family came from everywhere to be with us. Gary's family came from Utah. After all they had been through recently, and now this.

It was tough to walk through the church doors, but Lori, Gary, my boys, and I walked in together, made our way to the front, and took our seats. At the altar was a large picture of Brittany surrounded by flowers. They were all pink roses. The whole church was filled with pink roses. It was almost impossible not to burst into tears. I closed my eyes and imagined all the children coming to the front of the church and singing. This time, Brittany would be singing with them in spirit.

The Reverend got up and welcomed family and friends, and went on to say the things Reverends say about spirits returning home. Kat was supposed to speak next, but she was nowhere in sight. It wasn't like her to be late. We guessed she had been held up in traffic, so Barbara, and then Dawn, went ahead and spoke. They both gave beautiful tributes to Brittany and thanked us for giving them the opportunity to be a part of this experience. The calmness in their voices and the conviction of their beliefs gave us some comfort. Then, a man and woman, with the most angelic voices, sang *Somewhere over the Rainbow* and *The Rose*. As you can imagine, we were all moved to tears. I think Brittany was pleased to hear these songs and hoped we would find comfort in their messages.

As the last few lines of *The Rose* were being sung, in came Kat. She hurried up the aisle and slid in at the end of our row. She leaned forward, looked down the row toward us, and gave a little wave and smiled. When the song was over, Kat went up to the podium and gave another beautiful tribute to Brittany.

The service was moving and beautiful, but it seemed unreal. Lori, Gary, and I were just going through the motions of something we just couldn't comprehend. I remember thinking that if I just took a long nap; I would wake up and see her coloring at the kitchen table or riding her bike.

Friends and family gathered afterwards to share their hugs and words of comfort. It's hard for people to know what to say because they know it is impossible for them to take away the heartache. As those attending the service thinned out, Kat finally had the opportunity to tell us why she was late. She started by saying, "You won't believe what happened."

Our eyes grew big as we listened intently. She told us that on her way to the service, she got in an accident on the freeway that could have been deadly. Her car was hit so hard that it rolled over, but miraculously she ended up without a scratch. As the car was rolling, she saw Brittany in the passenger seat, rolling over with her. Brittany spoke to her, telling her that she would be fine and would make it to her service on time. When the tow truck arrived, she told the driver she was on her way to speak at a memorial service and asked if he could take her there right away. After hooking up her car, off they went, to the church.

This one really took us by surprise. Other than "Wow," I don't remember anyone saying too much. I think we were busy just taking it all in and wondering if Brittany was there, standing right beside us.

In the reception area, we had set up a table with pictures of Brittany and some of her favorite things. It was hard to set up and equally hard to take down. As we packed everything up, the reality that it was now truly over left us empty and unsure of what to do next. Even though we knew Brittany was no longer in pain and was in a happy and safe place, we were still hanging on to her. We knew it was time now to try our best to go back to our normal lives, but how do you do that when everything had changed so much?

Where Do We Go From Here?

Kat's incredible story and the comforting words spoken at the service helped ease our pain for the next few days. Brittany was now with God and surrounded by others in our family who had gone on before her. As I thought of where she might be, I pictured my father holding her in his lap and patting her on the knee, and, just as he did with me, telling her everything was as it should be. I knew he would take care of her. I'm sure Gary's sister Arlynne, who had been at her bedside in spirit, was there, as well. Envisioning them with her made it easier to fall asleep that night.

Friends and family who had traveled from afar had left for home to resume their normal lives. We now had to plan our lives without Brittany, but how would we fill the empty space that surrounded every breathing moment?

Would Erik wonder where she was, or was he too young to remember? She had loved her little brother and had given him so much attention.

Life was different now for our whole family, but especially for Lori and Gary. Over the next couple week, everyone had to think about life without Brittany and make their own decision about how they would move forward. Lori and Gary's lives and their relationship had been changing prior to his leaving for the Middle East and now this heartbreaking event would take its toll. The devastation from losing a child is too much for many couples, and it was too much for them. They decided to go their separate ways.

Lori took Erik and went to Salt Lake City where she attended massage school. Gary went to Fort Collins, Colorado, to recover emotionally and start anew. The road ahead would be long and hard for both of them.

Each of us now had to begin our own healing. The struggle to reclaim a serene and untroubled mind lay before us. Many tears would be shed in the days to come.

Some days were harder than others. At first, there was guilt for not realizing early on that Brittany had been so sick. I couldn't help thinking that if I had paid more attention, I would have seen a sign, something that could have saved her life. It broke my heart to know Lori and Gary were thinking the same way.

You do your best to carry on, but your heart gets stuck somewhere on the outside of reality. Questions about life, death, and the universe flood your brain because you want to understand what it all means. Loss of faith, confusion, and sadness can consume you. You know you don't want to feel this way for the rest of your life so you have to make a decision to do something about it. I knew it was time for me to try harder to make sense of things and pull myself together.

There is no detour around the pain. Grief is not just a feeling, but a process, and the only way past it is through it. It's a long, hard journey you have to make. Some find their peace quickly, while others search for years. Although time does heal, it's what you do with that time that makes a difference.

As I searched for answers, life carried on, and, as difficult as it was, I had to move along with it. One of the hardest things to deal with was all the "firsts" without your loved one. You have the first birthday, the first Christmas, and all the other holidays. If you have family traditions, you will experience them for the first time without that person. You will constantly hear and see things that remind you of them. No doubt about it, it's tough going.

The more determined I was to find peace, the harder I tried to have faith that the answers would come from God or this universal energy everyone talked about. I started reading books and listening to CDs, trying to find out what other people said about "the circle of life." It was time to figure out what I believed in and start living that belief.

Though I had experienced some unusual and moving things while Brittany was in the hospital, I wasn't completely convinced yet that they weren't coincidences. That bothered me. I knew what I needed to do was trust that as time went on, God would reveal something to me that would cause me to believe.

HEALING IS ABOUT EVERYONE

As I sat on the porch with a cup of tea, I wondered how I was going to release the emotional trauma that was still churning inside me. I felt like a lost soul trying to create a piece of heaven on earth without a clue how to do it. I wanted so much to believe things happen the way they're supposed to.

I began thinking back on all that had happened in the past months, trying to figure out what lessons I should have learned. I felt that every experience is supposed to teach us something, but this heavy feeling of sorrow had a way of blocking everything good from my mind. I was stuck and needed to find a way out.

What I really needed was to find a door that opened to a bright green patch of soft grass where I could tumble softly to the ground, take a deep breath, and sink into the comfort of God's arms. When your heart is breaking, human nature will push you to find something or someone that can take you to that patch of green grass. Sometimes, we just need a fresh start.

I had spent many hours wondering why God hadn't answered our prayers and why no one was able to heal Brittany. What was I missing? What didn't I understand?

As I sipped my tea, memories of our time in the hospital swirled in my head. The first thing I thought of was the pink rose I had seen in the garden. That rose bush had probably been there for years, but nevertheless, it was there for me to see on that day. Holding this vision in my mind, I could hear Kat saying, "Healing is not just about the sick, it's about everyone." At the time, her words went in one ear and out the other because they weren't what I wanted to hear. I had wanted the healing to be all about Brittany and no one else. My family and I were all so wrapped up in worry that we didn't notice the little things that were happening with everyone involved.

Perhaps I hadn't paid enough attention to the fact that so many people showed up at our time of need. Kat, Barbara, and Dawn seemed to come out of nowhere, right when we needed someone to lean on. Their life's work is about alleviating the suffering of others and moving them to a higher level of understanding.

I remembered the nurses describing a feeling of tranquility in the room whenever Kat, Barbara, or Dawn had been there. Considering what the staff of a children's hospital go through every day, I'm sure this was much needed healing for them, as well. I realized that by helping all of us, the three women had received an opportunity to use their gift, which moved them along their own life's path.

The Blue Blitz soccer team, Kaley, and her mother, Nancy, all had opened their hearts to us. The story about how they had helped our family had touched many. I wondered how many types of healings had resulted from the chain reaction of their generosity. The day Nancy and her friends had come to Brittany's room with rosaries in hand had brought peace to all of our hearts.

At the Sai Baba center, I remembered the surprised look on the clerk's face when Lori found the medallion. Maybe that moment gave the clerk what she needed to restore lost faith. You never know how your interactions with others will affect them.

As I recalled both the special and frightening moments that had taken place, I wondered how many others may have been strengthened in some way. I remembered the time we spent talking with the families of the other children in the hospital. In that scary place we had all shared, we had done our best to keep hope alive for everyone. From this, my own faith had been strengthened by each person I had encountered.

At the time, I don't think any of us fully realized how much love was moving to and from us all. It was like an invisible mesh of divine energy wrapping us all together. As God and His angels had watched us from their sacred places, they knew that in time we would understand these lessons of life and see that we had all, in some way, been touched and healed by His hands.

While she was in the hospital, our precious Brittany never cried or complained because she knew it was her time. We saw her as a little child, but she was a wise soul sent here to teach us to believe in something higher than ourselves and to trust there is a greater purpose for us all. She was taking the spiritual energy that was being sent to her from the healers and sending it back to us because she knew we needed it more.

When I finally understood that, the pain began to disappear and I could see her as a beautiful angel watching over us all. Never will a day go by that we don't wish she was here, but knowing she is only a breath away keeps her close and brings us a feeling of peace and contentment.

Chapter Four

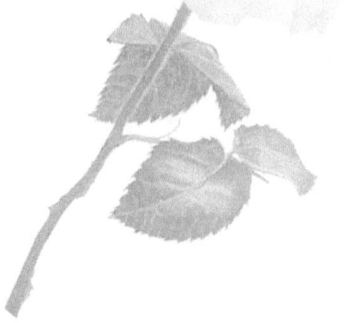

Learning to Heal

Miracles Happen

Now as I look back, I realize the many experiences I had while Brittany was sick and after she passed have all been moving me toward a higher level of spirituality, enabling me to have a better understanding of things we think are out of our reach. On that day, sitting in the sun on my porch, I had no sense of what the years ahead would be like. I had no idea they would be filled with messages from Brittany, giving me many heartwarming spiritual moments with her.

In the beginning, I accepted the thought that these experiences were not from Brittany, but were mere coincidences. However, in time, I came to accept and trust the messages she was sending. Once in a while, I asked for a message, but most of the time not. They would just come when she thought I need them the most. Once she saw that I recognized them and accepted them, they came more often. I still receive messages from her today.

The following stories are just a few examples of the many messages I've received and continue to receive. Some took place in only a minute or two, sometimes only seconds, but they illustrate my point. You might think the ones that happen quickly aren't profound enough to be meaningful, but let me tell you, when they happen, they have a huge impact. Every day, Brittany continues to build my faith and open my eyes a little wider to the wonders of Heaven.

If you feel you have received a message from a loved one, don't call it a coincidence. The key is to *believe it's possible* to receive one. Don't downplay these experiences, because no one on this earth can tell you it isn't exactly what you believe it to be. Give meaning to everything you receive from your angel. Make it a big deal. Don't let your angel down. Let their messages lift you up and warm your heart because that's exactly what they are meant to do.

Don't spend your time waiting for something extreme to take place. If you do, you will miss the most moving experiences of your life.

Miracles happen when we are open to believing they can.

THE "ONE-MINUTE ROSE"

My "To Do" list seemed to have more on it than I could do in a day. It always seemed to end up like that, so I just started with number one and did as much as I could.

With Saturday's chores behind me, I was ready to kick up my feet and just do nothing. It wasn't just my feet that felt tired. It was also my brain. I was worn out from trying to constantly push away a mixture of my own grief and that of my family's. A few months had passed and I was hoping by now I would be feeling somewhat better, but the pain . . . it just stays with you. I was pretending to be fine, but was still searching for the peace of mind I hoped would automatically take over at some point.

I lay back on my bed and asked the evening breeze to swirl around me and lift me up to where Brittany was so I could just feel her presence for a few moments. I wanted to see her sweet little face and hear her laughing freely or see her skipping along that golden road chasing a butterfly. I raised my hands toward the ceiling, thinking that if I concentrated hard enough, I would feel her fingers touch mine, even if just for a second.

I dozed off and before I knew it, I awoke to a new day. I went to the kitchen to make a cup of tea. As I put the pan of water on the stove, the clock caught my eye. It was eight-thirty. For some reason, the word "church" popped into my head. As the water heated, I began thinking about the church Dawn had introduced me to, the one where Brittany's service had been held.

Every time I had seen Dawn at the hospital, she had invited me to come on Sunday and always saved me a seat. I had gone a few times while Brittany was in the hospital, feeling more comfortable each time I went. I wanted to go every Sunday, but I had a hard time dealing with how the service began. It always began the same way. The younger kids would flow in from the back of the chapel and make their way to the front and sing to us in their little angelic voices. I would look around and watch the parents stretching their necks out as they tried to catch a glimpse of their child. Normally, I would get all wrapped up in the sweetness of the moment and probably stretch my neck out, too, trying to pick out the one I thought was the cutest. Instead, I struggled to hold back the tears because I couldn't help picturing Brittany up there singing with them.

I took my tea out onto the porch and started to plan the day, but I couldn't keep my train of thought. I kept seeing flashes of Dawn in the row near the back, on the right-hand side where she always sat.

Suddenly, I had an overwhelming feeling that I should get ready and go. I looked at my watch and figured if I hurried, I would make it with a few moments to spare. It felt odd to be so moved to do something this quickly without thinking about it further. I thought maybe God was calling me to go because He knew I needed some uplifting. I did enjoy going, but the kids . . . the kids will walk in and sing . . . and I would cry. After thinking about it some more, I decided not to go. As I tried to put it out of my mind, something stronger began pulling me in the direction of the church. I couldn't understand it, but I was curious to know why I was being pulled so hard, so I decided to go and find out.

As I drove, I had flashbacks of the day Brittany's service was held at this same church. I could see the sad faces of family and friends as they sat quietly with teary eyes. I remembered seeing dozens of pink roses filling the front of the church with a sweet picture of Brittany right in the center. The fragrance of the roses was still fresh in my mind. I remembered sitting with my family and hoping with all my heart that the words that were said that day would somehow lift our heartache. How could I walk into this church and not think of that day?

A terrible sadness suddenly came over me. Why risk emotional anguish when I didn't need to? It was all too much so I decided not to go.

All of a sudden, as I turned to head back home, I looked up at the sky, hoping to find the peace of God. There, right in front of me, was a beautiful set of sunbeams branching out from behind a big, white fluffy cloud. The rays of light were extremely bright and reached right into my car. Again, as had happened months before, I was deeply affected by what I was seeing. I quickly pulled to the side of the road and began to cry. There was a mixture of emotions that made it hard to figure out exactly what I was crying about, but whatever it was, I hoped I would come to understand it in time. As my chin rested gently on the steering wheel, I felt the warmth of the sun melt into my skin. The rays of sun seemed to be telling me there was an important reason to turn around and go back to church.

I wanted so much to believe there was something good in store for me if I went back. While sadness pushed me toward home, hope and faith persuaded me to gather up some courage, and headed back to the church.

I made it with ten minutes to spare. There at the front door was Reverend Don, who had spoken at Brittany's service. He was shaking hands and hugging people as they made their way into the church. I was afraid to walk closer. Would he remember me? As I stood on the front lawn watching people file in, flashbacks of Brittany's service filled my head again. I wasn't even in the church yet and already I was fighting back the tears as I thought of the kids coming in to sing. When will this be OK? When will I not feel so sad? I decided there was no way I could go inside.

Just as I was about to turn and walk away, the Reverend caught my eye. He smiled and began walking toward me. Oh boy, he did remember me. He reached out with both arms and pulled me in for a hug. It was a friendly, warm hug, one I needed more than I knew. My eyes got teary as he put his arm around my shoulder and walked me toward the entrance. A sensation of relief grabbed me by surprise. For the first time, contentment and joy seemed possible.

I looked over to the right, back section and there was Dawn in her usual place. I told the Reverend I was going to sit with her. He gave me a smile and a pat on the shoulder and nodded.

I walked to the side and waited to get Dawn's attention. She saw me right away and motioned for me to come and sit with her and her husband. It felt good to be there with her. There was something about her that allowed me to feel at peace. She was like an angel who knew me better than I knew myself.

There was barely enough time to get comfortable before the music started. In the corner of my eye, I saw the children starting to walk in. I kept telling myself, "Don't cry, don't cry."

A tear snuck out anyway and ran down my cheek. Dawn reached over and squeezed my hand. That, of course, brought another tear. As hard as I tried not to, I imagined Brittany standing there singing. My heart and mind had such a battle going on. My mind told me God was taking care of her, but my heart ached to have her there with me.

After a pleasant welcome from the Reverend, a woman stood up to give some announcements. Her first words were accompanied by a big smile as she said, "I know you all will be glad to hear that Ed Rivera and his wife are visiting today."

I could see by the reaction of many that this couple had been there before. Everyone seemed to know exactly why they had come. Dawn leaned over and explained that Ed Rivera had a thirty-minute program on TV where he showed people how to paint a rose in one minute. He called it "The One-Minute Rose." He and his wife traveled around the world helping churches raise money. You donate money and he paints you a rose. It was that simple. We were told he would be in the back of the reception area right after the service to paint a rose for those who wanted to make a donation.

My whole body tingled. I felt I was enclosed in a capsule of heavenly light where no one could see me, touch me, or speak to me. In that moment, I realized why I was there. Brittany had been the force that had pushed me into the car and hadn't let me turn back. I couldn't see her, hear her, or feel her breath on my neck, but I knew she was there with me.

The words and music of the service passed in a blur. I had no idea what the sermon was about. I was totally focused on how I was going to ask this man to paint a pink rose . . . without bursting into tears.

After the service, we all got up and started making our way out. Many people headed toward the reception area to make their donations and have their paintings done. I walked out with Dawn and her husband and thanked them for letting me sit with them. She pulled me aside and asked if I was going to get a painting. My throat burned as I held back the tears. It was impossible to speak so I just nodded yes. She gave me a hug and said she hoped to see me next Sunday.

A crowd of about twenty gathered for their paintings. If you weren't standing near the front, you couldn't watch as Ed Rivera painted. Since I was in no hurry, I sat down and patiently waited in the background. Over and over I rehearsed how I would ask for my rose.

It took about thirty minutes for the crowd to thin out. When only two people were left, I stood up and walked closer. I noticed how Ed's wife smiled as she handed him fresh paint and a clean brush. I thought of how they must enjoy doing this together and how wonderful it must be to share joy as you travel around the world. The radiance in their faces made it obvious they were sincerely grateful for the opportunity to serve in that manner.

The last person was now watching her rose being painted. I was next. Should I tell him why I wanted pink or just ask for pink? I knew I should just ask for pink, take my rose, and go home like everyone else, but it wasn't that easy. I knew Brittany was there, and she knew how special this moment was.

It was now my turn. As I stepped forward, I got choked up before saying even one word. Ed's wife reached over and touched my arm as he stood there smiling and waiting for me to regain my composure. They could see I had a special reason for this rose.

I took a deep breath and asked, "Can you paint two for me?" I had to get one for Lori, too. This would be a special gift.

"Of course I can," he answered. "What color would you like?"

"Pink, I would like them both to be pink," I answered with a slightly broken voice.

"Then pink it is," he said with a smile. "These must be special roses."

I nodded yes. I wanted to say more, but every time I started to speak, tears welled up in my eyes. It was obvious to both of them that deep emotions were tied to these roses. His wife was so sweet. She came over and gave me a hug and asked if I wanted to talk about it. I wanted to, but every time I started, tears came, and I couldn't speak.

His wife patiently waited to see if I was going to be able to tell my story. She didn't push it, but I knew she was hoping I would. I felt they were sincerely interested, so I took a deep breath and tried to tell an "in-a-nutshell" version. I explained what happened to Brittany, but even more moving to them was the story of how she brought me there that day.

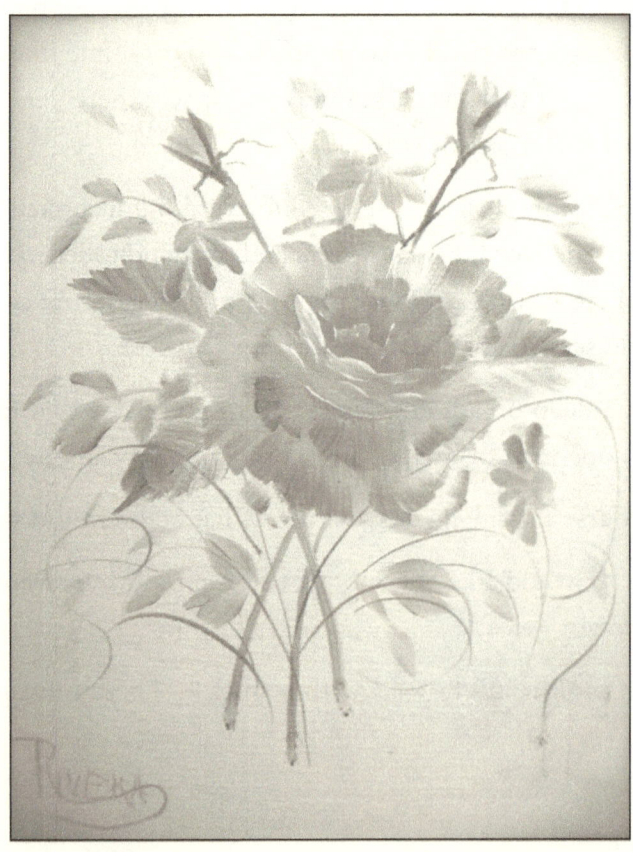

I watched as Ed painted each petal with ease and perfection. Little by little, the rose came to life. There was a chair close by, so I sat down so I could be at Brittany's level, just in case she was beside me.

Soon, he finished the second rose and propped it up to dry. Then came something I didn't expect. He looked me in the eyes and began telling me how they had lost their daughter years ago. As he spoke, his wife reached over and took his hand and smiled. There was no sign of emotion in his voice, but his eyes became wet. It was a sad, but beautiful, story. Even more beautiful was how their love and belief in God had brought them through their tragedy and sent them on a remarkable new journey of spreading joy all over the world.

It was surprising how connected we became in that moment. The entire day had been like a dream. We exchanged phone numbers and said we would keep in touch. They said I could call anytime if I needed to talk.

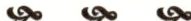

I couldn't wait to hand a painting of a beautiful pink rose to Lori and tell her about this incredible day. I knew she would agree that none of it had been a coincidence. I was overwhelmed by this experience and needed to go home and let it sink in.

I truly felt a door had opened that connected me to heaven and gave me a peek into the mysteries of the universe. I knew that something so profound might not happen every day, but I had a feeling it would happen again.

A Surprise In The Mail

A few months later, I got an unexpected envelope in my mailbox. It was from Florida. My brother lived there, but this wasn't from him. It was handwritten, so it seemed to be personal, but I couldn't think of anyone else I knew in Florida. I grew up there, but hadn't kept in touch with anyone other than my brother. There was no name on the return address, just the street, city, and state. Who could this be from? After opening it, I went straight to the end to see who signed it. To my surprise, it was signed, Ed Rivera. I thought maybe he and his wife were writing to let me know they would be in the area on their "One-Minute Rose" tour and would like to get together.

The letter began by asking how I was and by saying they hoped I was enjoying life and had found peace regarding the death of my granddaughter. I couldn't believe they had thought about me and had taken the time to write. I was hoping to read that they would be coming for a visit.

What I read in the next paragraph left me speechless. They had been so touched by my story that they had renamed the "One-Minute Rose" program. They were now calling it "Brittany's Rose." As I held the letter to my chest, tears ran down my face. I was so moved I could barely think. They had sincerely reached out to lift me up, but I had never imagined that I had lifted them up as well. This was a perfect example of the saying, "Love begins within and moves outward." Meeting them at the church that day had been God and the universe working their magic . . . doing what they do best.

I couldn't wait to tell Lori. Once again, I was amazed by how love takes its little threads and weaves us all together. Every story told connects more and more people in this circle of life. It just goes on and on.

TRUST YOUR ANGEL

When you lose a loved one, a part of your heart goes with them, and when a part is missing, your heart just doesn't beat the same. You struggle to keep faith and do your best to believe there is a purpose to all things. I had asked God to whisper in my ear and tell me how to heal this pain. I had even gone so far as to ask that He please tell me NOW.

God had said, "All right then, let Me see what I can do." So, I'd asked for an answer, right now, and for it to come by way of a whisper in my ear. Yes, that's exactly how I expected my answer to come, and that's where I got it wrong. While I was waiting for that whisper, I had missed my answer because it had come in a different way. God answers prayers in many ways and sometimes those answers come by way of our loved ones who have passed on.

It took a long time for me to understand this. As unusual things kept happening, I kept writing about them in my journal. In the beginning, I called them coincidences, but as time went on, I came to see that they were messages. Brittany had been trying her best all this time to let me know she was right beside me. Many of the answers I had been looking for were right in front of me on the pages of my journal. God had been answering my prayers all along.

If you are still seeking answers, let them come without any preconceived idea of how you should get them. I promise you, one day, out of the blue, you will hear or see something that will stop you in your tracks. It will be a message from God Himself, or your own sweet angel.

A Remarkable Moment

At times, it was still difficult to adjust to life without Brittany. I had to constantly remind myself that moving on didn't mean forgetting. It only meant that you have accepted the loss and are at peace with it.

I woke up this day with a strong need to talk to a friend . . . any friend. Flipping through my phone book, I looked for someone who could help me with whatever it was I must need. I wasn't even sure what that was, but had learned from experience it's good to reach out for help when you feel the need. As I turned page after page, no name jumped out at me. I thought, maybe I should just go see a movie.

I stretched out on my bed for a minute and closed my eyes, but I couldn't rest. The need to call someone persisted.

Again, I looked through my phone book. There, under the letter "C," I saw the name Cathleen. Some time ago, her name had been given to me as person who had strong spiritual beliefs and was able to help people whose loved ones had passed on. I had forgotten about her, but as I looked at her name, I was sure she was the one I should call. Maybe she could help me find the connection I wanted with Brittany.

It was Saturday, so I wasn't sure if she would be home, but she answered the phone. I explained how I had gotten her name and asked if she would have some time to talk with me. She said she and a few others were getting together Sunday morning and asked if I would like to join them. There was something in her voice that made me feel she knew I needed to be there. I can't explain it. I just felt it. I said yes without hesitating. It felt good to have somewhere to go with hopes of being uplifted. Something was pulling me, just like it did before, so again I was curious to find out why.

The following morning, I was on my way to a church to meet Cathleen. I had never been there before so I didn't know what they did at their service. I arrived about twenty minutes early, parked the car, and walked over to the church. When I walked into the entrance area, Cathleen greeted me with a smile. Immediately, a sense of calm came over me. I could see in her eyes that she had something to give. She introduced me to a few of the people who had already arrived and then showed me into a small chapel.

She said with a gentle smile, "It's just a small group, but I think you will be glad you came."

I suspected I would have a warm feeling when I walked in, and that's exactly how it was, quaint and peaceful. Since I didn't know anyone, I took a seat by myself in an empty row. I saw a man setting up a CD player in the front and assumed he would be playing music for the service. About fifteen people showed up, and they all seemed to know each other.

Cathleen began the service by asking that everyone be silent and welcome in the spirit. In that moment, I felt a part of this group and bowed my head along with the others and asked for the spirit to be with us. After a couple minutes, the man up front pushed a button on the CD player to start the music. As the melody began, my heart stopped and my eyes opened wide. I felt as though everyone was staring at me, but no one was. They all had their heads bowed and their eyes closed. I knew the first three beats of the song like the back of my hand. The song was *The Rose*. I wasn't expecting something so profound to happen. I was so moved, the tears just rolled down my face. I couldn't stop them.

An incredible feeling immediately moved through me. It felt as if part of my spirit stayed inside me and part came out and wrapped around my shoulders like a cape. I was in a warm, comfortable world of my own. I sat there with my head down, thinking, "Oh, Brittany, are you really here? I miss you so much." I kept my head bowed and my eyes closed as I waited for some kind of assurance that she was really there. It was only a matter of seconds before I saw her in my mind, smiling at me and saying, "Grandma, please believe that I am not gone. I am right here with you."

I sat without moving as the tears trickled down my face. As quickly as I wiped them away, more would come. I don't even remember what happened from that moment on. I know people talked and music played, but my mind was someplace else. That was a moment I would cherish forever.

When the service ended, I stood up and waited while Cathleen chatted with a few people. Before leaving, I wanted to thank her for inviting me and tell her what had happened. As I stood there, I noticed the man who had played the music was walking toward me.

I didn't want him to see that I had been crying, but there was no way to hide it. He walked up to me and said with a smile, "Welcome. I see you were moved by our service."

"Yes," I nodded, but didn't say why.

He put his hand on my shoulder and said, "I noticed the opening song seemed special to you. I saw it brought tears to your eyes."

"Yes," I replied. "It does have a special meaning." He continued to look at me, waiting to hear more, so I went on to tell him about Brittany and why *The Rose* meant so much to me.

He took my hands and looked me in the eyes and said, "Let me tell you what happened while I was driving here this morning. On the seat next to me was my notepad with a list of the music I was going to play. For some reason, I picked up my pencil and scratched out the opening song I had chosen and replaced it with *The Rose*.

I had no idea why I was compelled to do that, but I knew I would probably find out. Now I know why. You came here for a sign and that's exactly what you got."

I got a little chocked up as he gave me a well-needed hug. Just then, Cathleen appeared. The man smiled at her and then went on his way. As we walked out, I told her what had happened and thanked her for giving me a day I would remember forever.

She smiled and said, "There are no coincidences. You just shared a remarkable moment with your granddaughter. Isn't this why you came?" I was so surprised to hear this! How did she know? I nodded my head and smiled. She gave me a big hug and said, "In time, you will see that you don't have to try so hard to connect with her. All you have to do is focus on her spirit and you will see she is always thinking of you."

While driving home, I realized that these two complete strangers knew Brittany had led me to them. I followed Cathleen's advice and focused on Brittany's spirit. Suddenly it became clear to me that Brittany not only wanted me to have this experience with her, but she also wanted to let me know there are people who want to help others learn about how our spirits stay connected forever. Everything that had taken place throughout this entire experience was beginning to make a little more sense.

There Is No Distance Between Souls

Hundreds of books have been written about life and death, and I have read for hours, hoping to find that one special book that would take away the pain and explain everything.

People who write about life and death can only tell us what their own experiences have led them to believe. Some people believe each soul decides how and when they will leave this earth. They believe that we all have a purpose, and we will leave when we've learned what we came to learn, or when we have taught the lessons we came to teach. Some say there is a lesson to impart "on our way out" and we will "go out" in the manner we choose in order to impart that message.

Others say that when a love one dies, in order for them to move on and do "their work," we have to let them go. How does someone know we have to "let our loved ones go"? What exactly does "let them go" mean, anyway? I can't even read that phrase without feeling a hole in my heart. It always bothered me when someone said I was keeping Brittany from moving on and doing her work. I struggled for years thinking I was terrible for trying to keep her close to me.

I now know that you don't have to let go of your connection to the ones you love. It's OK to keep them close. In fact, it's actually impossible to sever the tie because there is no distance between souls. We are all a part of this universe and are all joined together for eternity.

SPIRITUAL CONNECTIONS

After Lori finished massage school, she moved back to California to work as a massage therapist. I was so happy to have her close by again. There were things I could share with her that I couldn't share with anyone else in the same way. She is still my rock.

I was looking forward to hearing stories about the different people that came for a message. She has told me that some clients lie still while being massaged without ever speaking, and some talk non-stop. Some clients tell some pretty interesting stories—she has heard strange stories, funny stories, and some stories that were spiritually moving.

Some clients are not only physically stressed, but also emotionally stressed. Lori has been blessed with the ability to connect with people through her gentle, kindhearted spirit and also through her touch. Many times during a massage, she has asked the person how they were doing, and they have broken down and poured out their feelings to her. Her understanding nature helps her heal both their body and spirit. All I can say is . . . she has a gift.

On one particular day, she had a new client named Hillary. After a quick hello and some friendly chit-chat, she got Hillary set up on the table, turned on some soothing music, and began the massage.

About halfway through, Hillary lifted her head and said, "Did you have a daughter who passed away?" Lori paused for a minute to recover from the sudden shock. "Yes, I did," she replied, as she continued massaging.

Hillary lifted her head again and said with a smile, "Sara says to tell you she's fine."

Lori was so stunned she didn't know how to react. She knew she couldn't stop and have a conversation, so she continued with the massage, but her mind was completely consumed with what the woman had just said. How did she know Lori had a daughter who passed away, and how did she know to call her Sara?

Hillary must have known what a statement like that would do to Lori. That's just not something you throw at someone unexpectedly. I probably would have fainted. Lori had another client coming in right after Hillary, so they didn't have time to talk much, but they did exchange phone numbers so they could get together later.

When Lori came home and told me what happened, I couldn't believe it. "You're kidding!" I said. "How did this woman know that? You never met or spoke to her before, right?"

"Mom," Lori said. "This was the first time I met her. I have no idea how she knew that. I was absolutely speechless and in shock. It seemed weird to continue the massage, but I didn't know what else to do."

"Lori," I asked. "Why do you think she got her name wrong and called her Sara?"

"Well, she didn't actually get it wrong. Brittany loved the name Sara. When she played, she sometimes pretended her name was Sara."

"Really," I said. "I didn't remember that. Why do you think she liked that name?"

"Well," Lori said, "One afternoon when we lived in Colorado and Brittany was three, Gary, Brittany, and I went out for a hike. We hiked all the way to the top of Henna Hunt Falls near Colorado Springs. As we came to this lake, Brittany suddenly stopped. She looked at me and said, "Do you remember when I was bigger than you and we drowned here? My name was Sara.""

Somewhat stunned, Lori had told Brittany she didn't remember. Did Brittany make it up or was she remembering a past life? Lori had read a lot about past lives, but what Brittany had said really threw her for a loop. Maybe they were together in another life. If you believe in reincarnation, I guess you wouldn't be surprised. If you don't, I'm not sure where to go with this. Some people believe we come back many times to learn or teach new lessons. Maybe this shouldn't be so hard to believe. After all, your soul entered your body when you were born, so why couldn't it enter another body at another time? I'm just keeping an open mind.

We still wondered how this woman knew to call her Sara, and how did she know she had passed away? We later found out that Hillary was a psychic to the stars . . . as in movie stars. She did readings and past-life regressions for famous people. She later told

Lori that she had been using her ability since she was a child, and because she had done it for so long, it didn't seem unusual to her. She forgot at times how shocking it could be to someone who hadn't experienced it before.

Although experiences like this are sometimes startling, they will strengthen your belief. Consider it a great blessing to have your loved ones remind you from time to time that they are not far from you. The more you open up to these kinds of experiences, the more they will happen, and the more you will feel at peace.

The Answers Will Come

The company I had been working for had filed bankruptcy, and soon I found myself looking for a new job. If you have ever gone through this, you know what a grueling process it is. Some people say, "Every time one door closes, another one opens," and I have learned many times that this is true. After much searching, I had an interview set up with a medical company. I knew the drill: dress nicely, stand up straight, look them in the eye while speaking, and be sure to give a firm handshake when saying hello. So, off I went with resume in hand to find my new employer.

After waiting patiently to be interviewed, a woman took me in to see the executive. He offered me a chair, so I sat down and got comfortable. I introduced myself, gave a nice handshake, and handed him my resume.

The first thing he asked was, "What have you been doing the last couple years?"

I asked, "Do you mean job-wise or personal?"

He answered, "Personal."

A bit surprised, I told him I had been working on a book.

He raised his eyebrows, smiled and asked, "What kind of book?"

I thought that since he worked in oncology and knew what struggles people go through, he might be interested in hearing about mine. As I spoke, he continued to ask more questions. He was quite interested in why I felt compelled to write a book, so I told him. I told him I felt my granddaughter had a purpose for being here, and I wanted to honor her life by writing about it. I told him that I had experienced many events that some might call coincidences, but that I had interpreted as messages from her. As long as he kept asking questions, I kept talking. I told him how I was struggling with knowing how to express my thoughts and still had questions about how to write them down.

He was impressed that I would take on a challenge like that and said he felt my book would be a success. It felt good to get this kind of encouragement, especially from someone like him. I had put the book project aside many times because I just didn't think I could do it, but the guilt of not completing it was always there, and after a while, I would pull it out again and begin where I had left off.

Next, we discussed the job and my qualifications. It seemed to be a good fit for both of us, and I felt the interview went well. When we finished, he walked me to the door, shook my hand and said he would contact me soon.

Having such a long, positive conversation with him about my book inspired me to dust it off and start working on it again. I was more excited about that than getting the job.

While walking to my car, I looked to the sky and told Brittany that I didn't think I could finish the book without her help. I promised her that if she would help me, I would start working on it again.

I got in my car, turned on the ignition, and on came the radio. A song was just beginning, and the first three beats stopped me cold. This song had been engraved in my brain and etched on my heart. The song was *The Rose*. I broke into tears and just sat there with my head leaning against the steering wheel.

I could feel Brittany sitting on my lap. I gave her a big hug and kiss and sat there for a few moments just holding her tight. I knew this was her way of saying, "Yes, Grandma, I will help you. I will be right there with you whenever you need me." I sat there for about fifteen minutes holding her tight in my arms.

When I got home, I sent an email to the man who had just interviewed me. I thanked him not only for the time he gave me, but for giving me a moment with my granddaughter.

He replied, "The greatest gift is to have faith that the answers will come."

Well, I didn't get that job, but as you can see, that particular interview had its own agenda.

Just Look Up

Many times we look toward heaven when we feel the need for something greater than ourselves to give us understanding, guidance, or comfort. As long as we have questions, we will never stop reaching out, whether we are praying, meditating, or doing something else we believe will bring us the strength or insight we're looking for. As we search, sometimes we find new places to get strength, places we never thought of. If what you've been doing doesn't seem to work anymore, it's time to search for something that will.

When Brittany was sick, the sky became my buddy as I drove to and from the hospital. When you see sunbeams dart down through clouds, do you look at them for longer than a few seconds? If not, you should. The sun and clouds create the most amazing pictures in the sky. I remember as a child thinking that if you could get right under one of those rays of light, you could feel heaven touching you, and I've carried that thought with me all my life.

Let me tell you about one morning when I was on the freeway driving to work. Ahead of me, there it was, the morning sun fanning its rays through the clouds straight down on the houses in the distance and the rolling hills to the east. Right at that moment, people were being touched by heaven. I wondered if something magical was happening to them and they didn't even know it.

I kept staring toward the place where the sunbeams touched down. As I drove, they seemed to move farther away, making it impossible to ever catch up with them and get directly under their light. All my life, I had chased sunbeams wondering if I would ever catch up with them. That frustrated me because I wanted to know if it was possible to feel heaven's touch. As I was absorbing the beauty of the moment, I realized something quite startling: the hood and dashboard of my car were glowing! I couldn't believe what had just happened. There I was . . . right under the rays of light! I think some people call that an "Ah-ha moment." I wanted to stop and stay there, soaking it all in as long as I could.

I couldn't help but wonder . . . . how many times I had stared at the sunbeams in the distance and never noticed they were also shining on me? How many times had I not noticed because I didn't recognize what was right in front of me? All this time, I had wished for something I thought I could never have. I wonder how often heaven touches us and we don't even realize it.

Three Pink Roses

We all have something we've latched on to somewhere along the way that reminds us of a loved one who has passed on. As you know by now, pink roses have a special place in the hearts of my family. If I made a list of all the places you might see a pink rose, it would be a long one. As a symbol of love, people use roses to celebrate many things, and of course they are beautiful in a garden. Pink roses are printed on everything from underwear to fine china and are not considered to be rare, but what makes our pink rose special is the meaning we've given it.

If you haven't done so already, you need to give special meaning to those things in your life that keep you connected to your loved ones. Memories are our greatest treasure.

Several years after Brittany's passing, Lori decided to move into a house behind the complex where we had been living. She wanted a backyard for Erik and her new son, Gage. Before she moved in, we went to check it out. After walking through the house, we went out on the back porch. We stood there looking at the yard discussing the possibilities for gardening and so on. Then, to our left, right next to the porch, we noticed a rose bush that had three fully bloomed roses on it, and they were pink. I never cease to get chills when these things happen. We looked at each other and smiled. We stepped down from the porch and stood in front of the rose bush.

"Look, Lori," I said. "Three pink roses to welcome you. There is one for you, one for Erik, and one for Gage." Our sweet Brittany, she uses pink roses to plant a seed of love and kindness with each one she sends. Our job is to nourish those seeds and watch them grow. Your job is to do the same with the seeds your loved one plants.

MAKE IT A BIG DEAL

For Christmas one year, I made DVDs of our family history. I didn't want our family memories to disappear, and of course Brittany was featured in what I was creating. Since this was a time-consuming project, I started early in the year. I gathered pictures, slides, and movies from all my family members. It was a lot of work, but I was excited to be doing it. Many items had to be sent out for processing so they could be transferred onto CDs that I could use on my computer. I had researched a few places where I could get all the media conversion done, but hadn't made a decision yet.

As I was leaving for work one morning, I noticed a large van in the parking lot right outside my apartment advertising this type of service. Wow . . . this was perfect, just what I was looking for, and it was right there in front of me. I wrote down the number from the side of the truck and called to set up an appointment.

I found out that the driver of the van lived in my complex and the next day before work, he came by my place to pick up all my slides. After writing out the order, he said, "Don't worry about a thing. All the people who work for us have been trained in their specialty and are professionals. The work on your family history project will be taken over by Brittany."

Whoa. I'm sure he wondered why I stared at him in silence. After a short pause, with exhilaration, I said, "Good. I know she will do a great job."

You may wonder why I make a big deal of these things. Well, it's because these things are a big deal. Why dismiss such a joyous feeling? In my heart, I have a special place for moments like this.

IT WAS JUST A PHONE CALL

At work that same day, we needed to call a vendor about ordering some parts for one of our customers. I had asked our buyer to make the call, but he was busy. So, I asked for the phone number in order to make the call myself. Right before dialing, I asked him if I should ask for anyone in particular. He said, "Yes. Ask for Brittany."

Whoa, again. I felt my eyes start to water. "OK," I said to myself. "You are at work. This is no time to burst into tears."

While walking back to my desk to make the call, I wondered why messages come in such strange ways. Maybe Brittany was just keeping me alert. I smiled as I thought of her watching me. I'm sure she was smiling back.

I dialed the number. The phone rang a couple times and then a girl answered.

"This is SW Direct. My name is Sara. Can I help you?"

Sara! Calm and collected or not, that one threw me a little. OK, I knew I was going to ask for Brittany, but someone named Sara answering startled me. Hearing Brittany's name twice in one day was surprising enough, but to hear the names Sara and Brittany both associated with one call brought me to a standstill.

"Stay calm and act professional," I said to myself, as I took a deep breath.

"Hi, Sara, can I please speak to Brittany?" Now, that was just strange.

"Sure," she said. "I'll connect you."

At that moment, everything around me shut down for a few seconds as I thanked my little angel for reaffirming the connection we share.

I know things like this are always open to interpretation, but for me, it was all a "Hello" from my little angel, Brittany. That is how she works. She knew I was involved in doing the family history project and just decided to give me a little inspiration.

Chapter Five

We All Heal Together

A Spiritual Concert

A few months ago, Lori and I went to a concert at the Center for Spiritual Living to see Snatam Kaur perform. She's an American singer and songwriter who tours the world as a peace activist. Her music is the kind that enters your heart and never leaves. Listening to her is truly a spiritual experience. The room only held about 100 people, so it was easy to feel like you were sitting amongst a large family. Anytime I am with my daughter in this type of atmosphere, it feels as though Brittany is with us.

Before the concert began, several women were passing out handmade bracelets. They were made of beautiful clear-cut beads of various colors and shapes, sort of like crystals. I took mine and thanked them for it. I didn't look at it too closely right then because the first song was beginning, and I was excited to finally see Snatam Kaur in person. Lori had given me some of her CDs, so I knew I was in for a treat.

Halfway through, during a short break, I reached into my purse and pulled out the bracelet to take a look. The clear, round stones were a mixture of lighter and darker shades of pink. Right in the center of the strand was a small pink rose. I don't know how many others may have also gotten a bracelet with a pink rose, but it didn't matter. I held it tight in my hand and said a little thank you to Brittany.

The purpose of Snatam Kaur's music is to bring spiritual energy into your soul. With Brittany's little rose in my hand as I listened, that's just what it did for me, and for Lori, too.

Sometimes They Just Surprise Us

This morning, I had to go pick up something at the pharmacy. When I got there, several people were in line, so I decided to look at some greeting cards while waiting. I walked over to a couple of tall racks, the kind that twirl around so you can see all the cards. As I was admiring the beautiful scenes of nature on some of them, something caught my attention. I felt compelled to turn my head to the left. When I did, right there, smack dab in front of my nose, was a card with a little angel on the front. Her hands were under her chin, and written on the card was the message, "I miss you."

It took my breath away. A rush of warmth went through me as I looked at the little angel and said, "I miss you, too."

Right under that card, was another colorful one that displayed a delightful garden of flowers. Almost at dead center was an old fashioned wheelbarrow filled with pink roses. I smiled to myself, and then my eyes were taken down to the next card just below that one. On the face of the third card was a brightly colored rainbow reaching across a beautiful blue sky. A rainbow has long been a symbol representing the beginning and end of life, and *Somewhere over the Rainbow* had been sung at Brittany's service.

Well, I'm sure you know I didn't just walk out of that store dry eyed saying, "Wow, what a coincidence." I know that Brittany has her own way of connecting with me, and sometimes in surprising ways. I see and feel that connection all the time.

Angel Light

Lori has a large circle of spiritually oriented friends. Through this group, she had met a woman whose son had been fighting leukemia for about a year. Many people, including Lori, prayed for him daily. Lori knew well the pain his mother was going through. There is only so much you can do to fight this disease and everything that could be done had been done. Hopes and prayers were constantly being sent to them. I would check with Lori every day to see how he was doing.

Soon the day came when we heard he had passed away. My heart went out to his family because I knew, as many of you know, the heartache you feel. Fortunately for his family, their strong beliefs were helping them through this tough time.

Earlier that day, Lori told me that she had told the boy's mother that she had asked Brittany to be there to welcome him home. That night, I had a dream that went like this:

I was at, what appeared to be, a family gathering. There was a very pleasant man there who had a grandson about five years old. All of a sudden, this little boy stood up and began to sing. I can't remember the name of the song, but it was a song about loving one another. He sang with a sweet little smile on his face and a sparkle in his eyes. His voice was pure and completely in tune. The song was the kind that lifts your spirits and makes you smile.

For some reason, the grandfather asked if the boy could spend the night with me, and I said yes. The next thing I knew, the little boy and I were lying in my bed. All the lights were out except my night light in the vanity area by the bathroom. The door to my room was open, letting the light in. I could tell the boy was scared to be away from home with someone he didn't really know. I pulled him close and we talked about things he liked to do. In a short time, he fell asleep.

During the night, he woke up crying softly, which woke me. Again, I pulled him close and asked what was wrong. He said he had to go to the bathroom, but was afraid. I could see his fear as he stared at the light coming through the door. I thought back to when I was little and remembered how scary it was to be in a dark place with only a small amount of light coming from around a corner. If you were afraid of the dark when you were young, you understand. Well, this is what was going through his mind. He wanted to go to the bathroom, but he had to walk toward the light first and this scared him because he didn't know what was around the corner.

In my softest and kindest voice, I said, "You don't need to be afraid. That's Angel Light. Angels watch over us while we sleep. If we have to get up in the night, they don't want us to be afraid or trip and fall. I'll walk with you and you can see how nice it feels to be in their light." As we walked into the light, he smiled, looked up at me and said, "I feel safe in the Angel Light."

When I woke up, I started to understand the dream. For Christmas, my friend Diane had given me a beautiful nightlight that has a porcelain square in front of the light bulb and is engraved with a fairy sitting on a branch, looking at the small ball of light she holds in her hands. When the light is turned on, it shines through the porcelain and wraps the most warm and peaceful glow around the fairy. I always think of Brittany when I look at it. This is the nightlight that was in my dream.

One way your special angel connects with you is through dreams. In this dream, the young boy represented the boy who had passed away, who now felt comfort from the Angel Light as Brittany reached for his hands and guided him home.

YOUR THOUGHTS CREATE YOUR WORLD

Your mind rules your world and the world as you know it is right inside your head. So, when someone says to you, "It's all in your head," just turn to them with a smile and say, "Yes, I know." Your thoughts become your life, so choose them wisely.

You can't always control everything that happens to you, but you can control how you interpret it and think about it. The challenge is to fill your mind only with thoughts that make you feel good and give life meaning. This is not always easy because there are many people and things surrounding you that constantly want to get in your way and disrupt the harmony in your life. The good news is . . . there are many angels that will help you along the way. If you want to know if that's true, just ask them. Once you have asked, all you need do is let their message in. It's really that simple.

Every time you experience something that could be called a "coincidence," recognize it's your angel answering a prayer. Your angel knows when you could use a little boost and will come to your rescue in the way they think best works for you.

There is one other sure thing in life besides death and taxes. It is this: You always get to decide how you are going to think about something. Yes, you get to do that. That means it's all up to you. No one can tell you how to think or how to feel. You do that all by yourself. It's not what happens around you that gives you peace of mind, it's what happens inside you.

MESSAGE ON A TRUCK

My brother, Jimmy, who lived in Florida, had been in the hospital for ten days and was now ready to be released. He was still having a hard time getting around so I went to Florida for a couple weeks to help him.

161

We had to get him set up in a new place so we had lots to do. He hadn't found an apartment yet, so that was our first task. The next morning we made our "To Do" list. It was much longer than we had anticipated. We had to find an apartment, furnish it, get kitchen supplies and groceries, transfer his mail, etc. We went nonstop every day. Each night we would cross off what we had done and make a fresh list for the following morning.

We were together constantly so we had a lot of time to talk. The last time I was in Florida was when our father passed away, so the first night, we talked about our childhood and how much we missed our dad. That started Jimmy thinking, and he often asked, "Do you think Dad and Brittany can see what we're doing and are proud of us?"

Each time I answered back with a smile, "Of course they can see us, and they are very proud."

One day he asked in a curious voice, "How do you know they can see us?"

"Well," I said. "I know because I get little signs now and then that tell me they can."

"What kind of signs?" he asked.

I told him about the things that had happened to me that made me believe in what I was telling him. He agreed it was possible, but I could see he was still questioning it.

The last day I was there, we were driving down the highway. Ahead of me was a large truck. I tried to pass it, but too many cars were coming so I stayed behind it. As the traffic slowed for a red light, we pulled close up behind the truck. It was a big box-like truck with no writing at all anywhere on the rear, but something caught my eye in the top right corner. I looked up, and there was a pink rose. You would never expect to see something delicate like that on an old truck like this one. It wasn't a flower delivery truck or anything like that. It was just an old box truck with nothing painted on it anywhere . . . except for one pink rose on the back.

"Jimmy," I said. "Look at the top right corner on the back of this truck."

He looked up, and then he looked at me. He didn't say anything, but I could tell his mind was in deep thought. He just shook his head and smiled.

"That's how I know, Jimmy."

WE ALL HEAL TOGETHER

Life is about people, and that will never change. Remember, others going through their own healing process will want to reach out to you in your time of need because they understand what you are going through. Let them help you, for by doing so you will be helping them heal, as well. God will use their hands to reach out to you, and your hands to reach back to them.

Through all the many people who came into our lives during Brittany's illness, we got an "up close and personal" taste of love in its purest form. This burned an everlasting impression on our hearts and inspired us to reach out to others.

Have you ever noticed that no matter where in the world you may travel, a hug is still a hug, and the feelings we share when we hug another person are always the same? Words are never needed.

To this day, I continue to receive assurance from my little angel that we are all bound together forever. If our departed ones could appear to us with a message, it might be something like this:

> *"I have not left you. I am with you every day. I am*
> *at peace and surrounded by the light of love. I send you*
> *this love in the shining sunbeams that warm your day. Just*
> *believe . . . and you will feel their warmth. Please don't cry*
> *because that makes me sad. Seeing you smile makes me*
> *happy. If you close your eyes, you will feel my arms around*
> *you. I miss you too, and will be waiting for you because our*
> *life together has not ended. I love you so much."*

You will find there is always a ripple effect to acts of compassion and kindness because they touch the part of our hearts that is filled with unconditional love. This is how love spreads throughout the world and benefits everyone.

A MOST PRECIOUS GIFT

I had a new job that I loved, a great boss, and I was doing work I felt qualified to do. It was a win-win situation, and I was happy.

I didn't like going out for lunch, so I got my lunch from a woman named Anne who brought food by every day. She would knock on our door to let us know she was there. Those of us who wanted to buy something would come out and nose through her cooler to see what looked good. She was easy to get to know, and after several weeks, we were talking as if we were best friends. Finally, in one of our conversations, it came up that her daughter had been battling leukemia. This led to me to tell her about Brittany. Because we had both experienced the same struggle, from that point on we shared a special bond.

I'll never forget what Anne did for me on Mother's Day. Before going outside to get a sandwich, I grabbed the Mother's Day card I bought for her. We had become close enough friends that doing special things like that was more than appropriate. Through our discussions earlier, it had come out that her mother loved pink roses too. With a smile, I handed her the card, which had pink roses on it. She was touched that I would think of her. We both got teary-eyed as we hugged.

She quickly said, "Watch the cooler for a minute, I'll be right back." I stood by the cooler and watched as she went to get something from her car. As she approached, I could see a vase with pink roses in it.

As she handed it to me, she said, "There are three roses. They represent you, your daughter, and Brittany." I couldn't get over how sweet and caring that was. We hugged again and shared a few tears as I thanked her for this thoughtful gift.

Every day she would come and knock on our door. Whoever opened it would holler through the office that the "lunch lady" was there. She was the "lunch lady" to everyone else, but to me, she was Anne, my special friend with whom I could share all that I had experienced since Brittany passed on.

About four months later, Anne told me her mother had passed away and that she had to clean out her mother's house and get things in order. I knew how hard that was and offered my support. A few weeks later she brought me a box covered in pink wrapping. The warm smile on her face told me it was something special. I watched as she opened the box and pushed back the tissue that kept the gift safe. She reached in and pulled out a pink ceramic rose, about two inches in diameter with a long green stem. Of course, my eyes teared up.

As she handed it to me she said, "This is for you. It belonged to my mother. While I was cleaning her house, I came across it and for some reason I knew I was supposed to give it to you."

I was quite moved by the gift. I thanked her and gave her a big hug, and she went on her way. As I was walking back to my desk, a vision popped into my head. Because the vision appeared so quickly, I knew it was something to pay attention to, and I suddenly understood why Anne thought she should give the ceramic rose to me.

I know Brittany knew Anne and I were sharing our most precious thoughts because in my vision, Brittany was helping Anne's mother move into the spirit world. I saw their hands meet, and I saw them smile at each other. I believe Anne's mother sent a message to Anne saying, "This sweet little spirit, named Brittany, just welcomed me home. When you find my ceramic rose, will you please give it to her grandmother?"

When I took the rose home, I put it on my desk by Brittany's picture. As I sat there looking at it, I suddenly realized this rose with its long stem was identical to the rose we had put on the front of the program for Brittany's memorial service. I sat there in amazement for a few minutes. Experiences like this take your mind to a faraway place.

When I looked over at Brittany's picture, I could sense her eyes looking directly at me. The picture was the last one I had taken of her. Back when I took this picture, film was taken to a shop to be developed, and you never knew for sure what you had until you picked it up. I had dropped the film off right before Brittany went into the hospital. Later I had picked up the finished photos, but with all the commotion that followed, the packet of pictures sat on my dresser for months without being opened.

I finally opened the envelope a few weeks after Brittany's service. The picture that is now on my desk was the first one I saw. It had immediately brought me to tears. I wanted to jump right into that picture and hug Brittany tight. In the picture, one hand holds her brother Erik so he won't fall, while her other hand is up in the air as if she were waving goodbye. Her eyes sparkle and she has the smile of an angel.

To this day, the rose Anne gave me still lies on my desk next to that very special picture of Brittany.

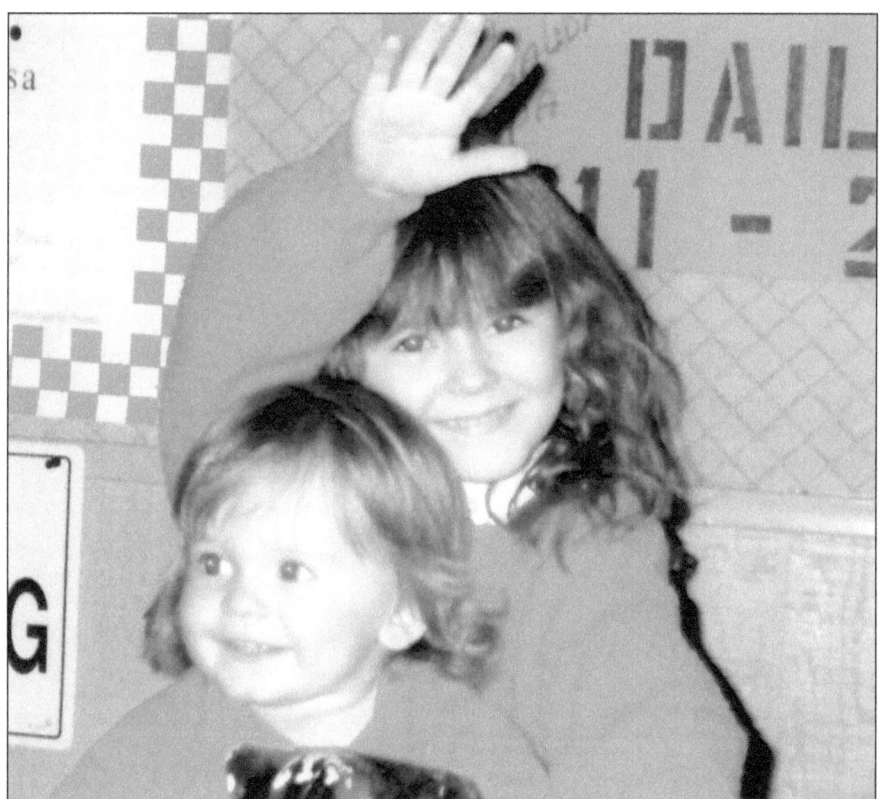

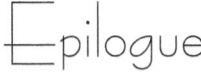Epilogue

The Disneyland Carousel—Brittany's rose

If you ever go to Disneyland in Anaheim, California, be sure to visit the King Arthur Carousel. There you will find a unique tribute to Brittany. Lori's husband, Rick Temple, an artist for Disney, dedicated one of the carousel horses in her honor. On its right shoulder, Brittany's horse has a pink ornate flower with leaves painted gold and trimmed with burgundy. Her horse, identified by the initials BR on the saddle blanket, is appropriately named Brittany's Rose. There is also a horse dedicated to Lori. Lori's horse, Lori Lyn, with the initials LL, and Brittany's horse are side-by-side on the carousel.

I Picked This Rose for You

I wanted Lori to read this book before I published it. It was hard for her, but she agreed to do it. As she got comfortable in her living room and began reading, there was a knock on her door. When she opened it, one of the little neighbor girls was standing there. In the girl's hand was a pink rose, one she had picked from someone's garden. Her big eyes sparkled as she said, "I picked this for you."

Let me remind you how this story began. It began with Brittany sneaking into our house with two pink roses she had picked from a neighbor's yard. She had given one rose to me and one to my daughter.

The neighbor girl knocking on Lori's door while she was reading this book, and then handing her a pink rose, was not just a coincidence. It was a message from our sweet little angel saying, "As always, I am right here with you."

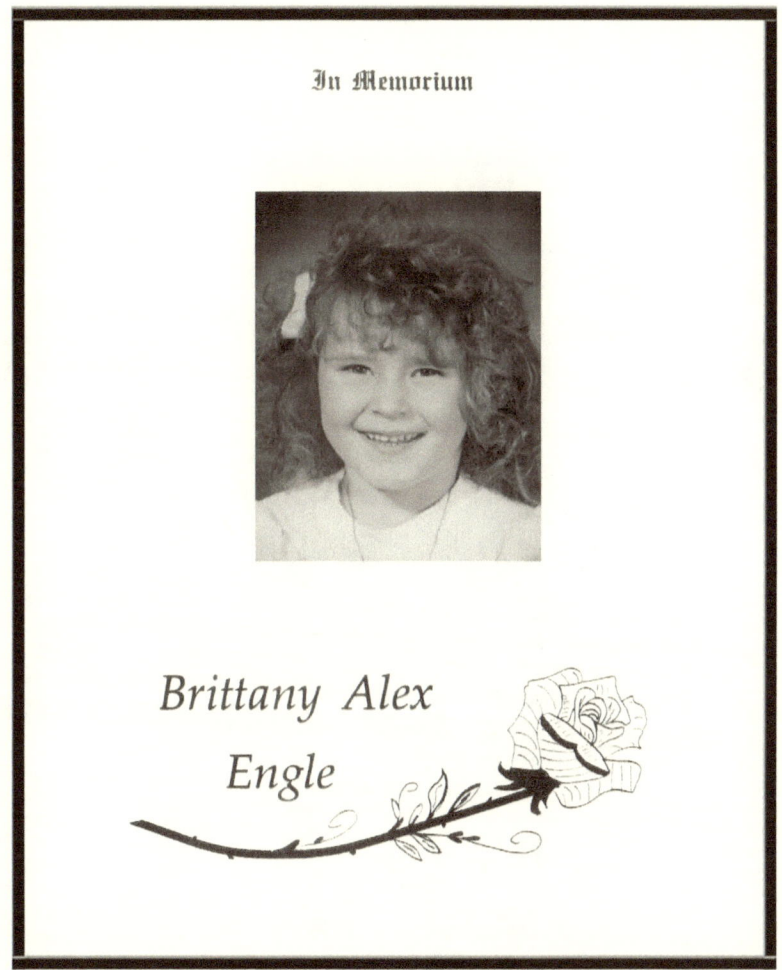

In Memorium

Brittany Alex Engle

A rose once grew where all could see, sheltered beside a garden wall.

As the days passed swiftly by, it spread its branches straight and tall.

One day a beam of light shone through a crevice that had opened wide.

The rose bent gently toward its warmth then passed beyond to the other side.

Now, as you feel its loss, be comforted, the rose blooms there.

Its beauty even greater now, nurtured by God's own loving care.

Author Unknown

To Do List

My "To Do" list has been redesigned a bit over the years. Life's priorities have changed as have the importance I have given them. This list was first designed when I was struggling to find peace and focuses on things that were helpful to me as I did my best to get through the grieving process. Even though I am finally at peace, I still use this list.

I remember thinking that if I started living my life as a happy person again, Brittany might think I didn't care about her anymore. I thought staying sad would prove to her how much I missed her. It took writing this book for me to understand that what makes our loved ones smile is seeing us enjoying life. They will always know how much we miss them, so we need to stop worrying about that. If you are still struggling, it's time to change things a bit and put a smile on your face and your angel's.

Here's a list you can try. This is what works for me. I keep it pinned up where I can see it every day. This is just a place to begin. What I've written could be expanded on quite a bit. If one part seems to have more of an impact on you, expand it or change it and see what you come up with.

- **Take Care of Yourself**

- **Embrace the Goodness that Surrounds You**

- **Do Something Nice for Someone**

- **Weed Your Garden**

- **Create a Gratitude List**

- **Look Up**

- **Just Believe**

Take Care of Yourself

If you aren't feeling good physically, it will be hard to take care of yourself spiritually and emotionally. Do your best to eat right, get plenty of rest and try to throw in a little exercise of some kind each day. Feeling physically well will clear you mind and help you tremendously in your other efforts.

Embrace the Goodness That Surrounds You

Accept the kindness of others as their gift to you. Easing heartache is not a simple task for anyone, so know that they are doing the best they can. Let the warmth of their kindheartedness wrap around you and lift you up.

Take a walk in the mountains, a stroll on the beach, or swing in a swing in the neighborhood park and enjoy the childlike feeling you experience. Getting close to nature is a great way to help you focus on the wonders of the world you are still a part of. Watch the sun rise or set, and let the beauty of the moment mesmerize you.

Ask a small child what he thinks is the most beautiful thing in the world, and watch the expression on his sweet little face as he tells you.

Pick some flowers, and study the pattern of their colors. It's amazing how nature repeats, without fail, its extraordinary designs in all living things.

<u>Remember</u>: Love from others is the greatest gift of goodness we can ever embrace.

DO SOMETHING NICE FOR SOMEONE

I'm sure you've heard it said many times that when you are down and out and want to feel better, you should do something nice for someone. It can be as simple as giving your time and attention, or even just a smile. You can be an angel in disguise for someone else. No matter how simple or elaborate it may be, it always works. When you give, you always receive.

Last year, I had a truly heartwarming experience that I would like to share with you. I decided to get serious about finishing this book, so I signed up for an online writing class. I learned a lot in the class, but one assignment in particular helped me realize the importance of our connection to other people.

Our instructor asked us to pick a color, tell why we picked it, describe it, and tell how it made us feel. Once I started working on the assignment, I realized this was much harder than I had anticipated.

When someone asks me what my favorite color is, the word "blue" rolls out without hesitation. I have never wondered why I love that color. I just know I do. Maybe it began with my father's blue eyes. His eyes had a gleam of kindness that made me feel safe because he always understood how I felt. Maybe God gave us each a different "favorite color" to make sure all colors would be noticed.

Our instructor told us that once everyone had finished the assignment, she would tell us why she had us do it. Knowing there was a special reason for this assignment made us all work harder at making it an example of our best writing. Once everyone had completed the assignment, we watched every day for a posting from our instructor.

Finally, her posting was there. She told us she had a dear friend who was blind, and every year she had her students complete this assignment so she could read what they had written to her friend. Chills ran through my whole body when I read that. What an amazing thing to do for someone, and we got to be a part of it.

Each person's assignment was posted on the website for everyone to read. I've never seen colors come so alive and have such extraordinary meanings attached to them.

After reading our assignments to her friend, she wrote back and gave us a vivid picture of the expressions on her friend's face as she listened intently to these beautiful works of art the class had created.

This was one of the most exhilarating experiences I've ever had. It was clear by the comments posted by the class members that the same chill ran through each of us as we realized the magnitude of the gifts we had given to this blind woman. This time, we were the angels in disguise.

I think everyone should do this assignment. You will be surprised how it makes you feel.

<u>Keep in mind</u>: People won't always remember everything you do and say, but they will always remember how you made them feel.

WEED YOUR GARDEN

The garden I'm referring to is the one in your head. Find a quiet place where you will be undisturbed. Start by doing some deep breathing. This is great way to clear your mind. Take a deep breath in through your nose and hold it for about five seconds. Then, blow it out through your mouth. Do this about ten times. It will help put you in a relaxed state. Some soft music would be a pleasant addition to this process.

Once you are relaxed a bit, you need to create a plan for weeding your garden of the things that make you sad. Making a list of the things you want to get rid of is a good way to get them out of your head. It's easier to focus on something when you can see it on paper. Your list can include things like old habits, old ways of thinking, and negative people.

Making a list is only the beginning. Next, you need to create a plan for ridding yourself of these bad weeds. Some people burn their list after they create it. As the flames carry the ashes up and away, they visualize negative thoughts leaving their life. You can also take one idea at a time and write out the steps you need to take to make a change. This will require some thought, so take your time.

When your mind is occupied with sadness, it's difficult to receive messages from your loved ones or to get any other type of inspiration. As you work to weed the garden and make positive changes in your life, you need to open your mind and your heart and let healing in; healing that affects your soul. As you let healing in, your emotional health will get back on track. This will help to open your connection to your loved ones and to God.

Remember: You are creating a new beginning.

CREATE A GRATITUDE LIST

When your world crashes down on you, it can become easy to feel there is nothing to be grateful for. The sadness of your loss can keep you feeling overwhelmed and unhappy for quite some time, if you let it. But, you are still a part of life, and you need to keep on living. One way to lift your spirits is to make a list of the things you are grateful for. Know there is still goodness to be had.

When you make your gratitude list, don't be too general and write things like family, friends, job, etc. Of course, our family and friends are absolutely one of our primary sources of joy, but what I'm asking you to do is be specific. We are working on emotional healing, so let your feelings be a part of this exercise. Go deeper and ask yourself what it is about these people, places, or things that make you grateful to have them in your life.

<u>Remember</u>: Don't wait for others to make you happy. Choose to be happy. Practice taking happiness with you wherever you go. The more you practice this, the faster you will feel happiness making its way back into your life.

LOOK UP

Sometimes, "up" is where we look for hope and inspiration. Other times, it could be we just want to feel the freedom of a wide-open space. No matter what time of day or night, the beauties of the sky can overwhelm us. Yes, there are scientific reasons for why the sky is blue, why clouds form, and why we are blessed with the extraordinary Northern Lights; but, nevertheless, these are God's creations.

Each sunrise and sunset allows you to see astounding images of God's handiwork. Along with their beauty, they bring a peaceful balance between mind and spirit. How long has it been since you laid on your back and watched the clouds form animals and silly faces? If you haven't done it in a while, you should. At times, you can see sunbeams shooting to the ground, painting exhilarating pictures.

At night, you can be amazed by all the twinkling stars and be filled with wonder about how many millions there really are. Think of how breathtaking it must be for astronauts to witness the cosmos from a perspective we can only imagine.

I look up because this is where I find inspiration that I can't find any other way. If the sky could talk, it would probably say something like this:

"When you walk outside today, just look up. You'll see me there. I have painted an electrifying canvas that surrounds your world and everything in it. I have the power to lift you up and take you as far as your imagination can reach. I penetrate your soul every day and continually open doors to all that is possible. All you know of life is protected by me and I hold the secrets to what lies beyond.

I am a blue diamond brilliantly cut with the ability to radiate my color back to you, filling you with the astounding force of life. I represent the essence of all the forms of life, and through my baby blues, I send to you my feelings of deep affection."

If you look at the sky with this message in mind, you will, without a doubt, find yourself sailing away on a cloud or swinging on a star and bringing moonbeams home in a jar. In these moments, you can feel the power of God's love. It's therapy for the soul.

Keep in mind: Once you open up and allow the beauty of the sky to come in, you will feel lighter and lifted up.

Just Believe

When we are emotionally broken, it can become easy for us to doubt our own feelings as we try to sort out all the things we've heard and read about the mysteries of life. The opinion of others, especially people we look up to, may also add to this feeling of doubt as they try to persuade us toward their way of thinking. As hard as it may be to sort through, we need this information to help us figure things out.

Learning to truly believe in something may take some soul searching. To receive answers to questions that lie heavy on our minds, it's important that we take time to sit quietly and dig deep into our own soul and learn to trust our gut feelings. Don't try to hurry this process, because if you do, you will find yourself having to start over.

Each person will come to believe what feels good to them based on their own life experiences. We each have to find our own way. No one has to agree with you, nor do you have to justify or prove your belief to anyone.

During your time of loss, there are many things you may wonder about. Maybe you want to believe your loved one is not gone forever. Maybe you want to know whether you can communicate with them. Maybe you are still not sure if God or heaven exists.

Is believing the same as having faith? Some will answer yes to that question, but I think faith leads to belief. Faith is trusting in something you have no proof of, but when you truly believe, you accept something as truth and you no longer question it.

I've listened to many seminars and read many books about "getting what you want." In essence, they all say that if you want something bad enough, you'll find a way to get it, but I don't think it's the level of *want* that stops us from getting to a place of belief. I think what really holds us back is being able to **truly believe something is possible**.

So, how do we get to that point of truly believing? Here are some things to think about.

1. <u>What do you believe in</u>? If you are already content with what you believe in, you will not be challenged with figuring this out. If you are still wondering, ask yourself what it is you wish you believed in. What one idea, if you could truly believe in it, would put your mind at peace? There may be more than one, so make a list. Once you pinpoint what idea is keeping you sad, you have a place to start.

2. <u>What is keeping you from believing?</u> Many people think it's fine to just have faith and not know the answer to anything because they don't think it matters. If you are still struggling, it does matter because you want to have peace of mind. So, what's holding you back? Perhaps what you want to believe in doesn't seem at all possible. Maybe you're afraid your family will disown you if you believe something that goes against what your parents taught you growing up. Maybe you are just afraid to believe. That might sound strange, but if the mysteries of life and life on the other side were to open up to you, would it change you? What would you do differently if you had all this knowledge? Once you figure out what is holding

you back, let it go, and open yourself up to accepting a new way of thinking.

3. Send your wish out. Ask for what you want and then release it out to God, the Universe, Heaven, whatever you call the place or person you feel holds divine power. If you have never done this before, it will take some faith on your part. Even if you don't believe this will work, just do it.

4. Stay open to receiving and trust in what you receive. This is the most important part of this process. In the beginning, you may call many of your experiences a coincidence, just as I did. You may want something you absolutely cannot question at all, like a vision. Because of that, you may not trust your experiences to be messages because they will have come in a way you didn't expect. It's also possible that one day you may see something, hear something, or just out of the blue have an incredible feeling of peace that erases all doubt. The important thing is to remember not to have a preconceived idea of how your answer will come because they will come in many different ways, ways you never thought of.

5. Believe doubt will fade with time. You will probably have to receive a message from God or your loved one a number of times before you truly believe it. You need to trust long enough to develop this new belief. Old habits of thought need to be broken. Trust that doubt will fade as you continue to give meaning to these events that move your soul. Once you accept the messages as real and not products of your imagination, a new world will open up to you and you will be at peace.

Always keep in mind that when we lose a loved one, it's easy to get stuck in the heartache for a long time, but the longer we are sad, the longer they are sad for us. We still have a life to live, and our loved ones want us to be happy.

Final thoughts

It hasn't been easy for me, but I never stopped believing I would find peace. You should never stop either. If you are still searching, don't stop until you find your happiness. It's right there waiting for you.

I'm so proud of my daughter, Lori, for listening to the lessons this experience brought. Her life is devoted to helping others learn how to live a long and healthy life filled with happiness. She's a massage therapist, a yoga and fitness instructor, and a raw foods instructor, and health counselor. She has a loving, kind heart and arms that will reach for miles to pull you in.

I'm also proud of Brittany's dad, Gary. He suffered many heartbreaking moments in his life that at one time, led him down a path of darkness, but he never gave up. Because of his strong will and the help of some wonderful people, he now has a life filled with happiness and success.

While Lori and Gary are no longer together, they still keep in touch. They each have found their own way to give back and do their part to make this world a better place.

Always believe in the goodness of life and know that your connection to all that is, and ever was, will never be broken. A joyful and content life is yours for the taking. Just reach out and grab hold. A warm hand will always meet you half way . . . the hand of your angel.

Memories are never meant to leave the heart because they are the most sought-after treasures. May you be blessed with time to enjoy your family and friends, and all the beauties of nature that God has put here for you.

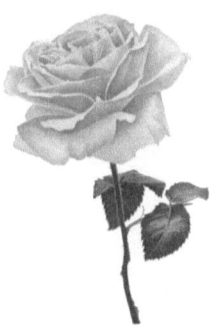

May God Be With You Everywhere

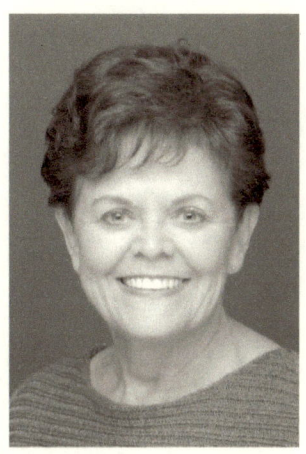

Mary Jane Clayton

is a writer and illustrator who lives in Southern California with her children and grandchildren.

She continues to share her story with others who are stuck in the grieving process in hopes of helping them find peace.

You may contact the author at:

mjclayton2003@aol.com

www.brittanysrose.com